A GOOD NIGHT'S

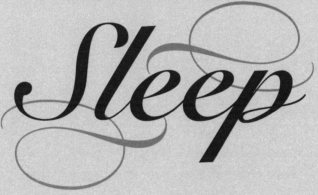

Sleep

A GOOD NIGHT'S

Sleep

Meir Kryger, MD

with

The National Sleep Foundation

METRO BOOKS
NEW YORK

This 2009 edition published by Metro Books.

This book is part of *A Good Night's Sleep* kit and is not to be sold separately.

Metro Books
122 Fifth Avenue
New York, NY 10011

ISBN-13: 978-1-4351-1168-4

Printed and bound in China

1 3 5 7 9 10 8 6 4 2

DISCLAIMER

WHILE THE PUBLISHER BELIEVES the information used in creating this book to be reliable, the medical field changes rapidly and there are new developments almost daily. The publisher cannot guarantee the accuracy, adequacy, or the completeness of the information contained in this book and must disclaim all warranties, expressed or implied, regarding the information. The publisher also cannot assume any responsibility for use of this book, and any use by a reader is at the reader's own risk. This book is not intended to be a substitute for professional medical advice, and any user of this book should always check with a licensed physician before adopting any particular course of treatment.

It is strongly recommended that if the reader has a sleep problem, they should not attempt to diagnose or treat themselves, but should always bring the problem to the attention of a doctor. Some of the treatments mentioned here were originally released to treat other conditions, and thus some of them are used "off label." Always consult your doctor about any medications you may be prescribed, and under no circumstances should a person use prescription medicines prescribed to someone else. The items included in this kit are not recommended for the treatment of any disease, and the reader should consult a doctor for any sleep disorders.

Acknowledgments

I WOULD LIKE TO THANK the fellow National Sleep Foundation (NSF) Board members, especially Dr. Jerry Kram for his expertise in developing several chapters and Dr. Amy Wolfson for her careful critique of the entire manuscript. I would also like to thank NSF staff members Colleen Cancio, Jessica Steinitz, and Michele Wagner for their assistance in the drafting of certain sections, editing, and fact checking. I would like to thank Kevin Ullrich and Christine Heun for the design, and finally, I would like to thank Devorah Klein of Barnes & Noble, Inc. for her superb editing skills and for pulling it all together.

About the Authors

MEIR H. KRYGER, MD, FRCPC is chairman of the board of directors of the National Sleep Foundation and past president of the American Academy of Sleep Medicine and the Canadian Sleep Society. He is currently Director of Sleep Medicine Research and Education at Gaylord Hospital in Connecticut and Clinical Professor of Medicine of the University of Connecticut. His research has spanned sleep breathing disorders, neurological disorders affecting sleep of both children and adults, and sleep problems in women. He is the chief editor of the main textbook used in sleep medicine, *The Principles and Practice of Sleep Medicine*, now in its fifth edition, and is the author of *A Woman's Guide to Sleep Disorders*. He was the 1996 recipient of the William C. Dement Award for Academic Achievement in sleep medicine.

THE NATIONAL SLEEP FOUNDATION is an independent nonprofit 501(C)3 organization dedicated to improving public health and safety by achieving understanding of sleep and sleep disorders, and by supporting sleep-related education and research. Visit NSF at www.sleepfoundation.org.

CONTENTS

Preface 10

Foreword 12

CHAPTER 1: The Science of Sleep 15

CHAPTER 2: Assessing Your Sleep Disorder 27

CHAPTER 3: Sleep Disorders 41

CHAPTER 4: Travel, Shift Work, and Your Personal Body Clock 75

CHAPTER 5: Children and Sleep 91

CHAPTER 6: Sleep and Aging 103

CHAPTER 7: Sleeping Pills, Medications, and Herbal Remedies 115

CHAPTER 8: Tips for Better Sleep 139

Resources 157

Index 161

Preface

Sleep.

Most people never think about sleep. They go to bed, shut their eyes, and drift off, and then wake up alert and in a great mood, ready to conquer the day.

Sleep.

For some it is a treasure that washes away the stresses of the day.

Sleep.

Some consider it a waste of time, interfering with the ability to earn more or to do more or to play more.

Sleep.

For some the night is a time of great distress. Sleep may not come easily or may not come at all. For others, it is when nightmares and demons call or when normal activities like breathing become abnormal and can endanger one's life.

Sleep.

When someone's brain has not had enough sleep, it will crave it. Sleep may come suddenly in people, and depending on what they are doing, may endanger them and those around them.

Sleep.

It has been estimated that about 50 million Americans have sleep problems. For some it is only once in a while. For some it is every night. For some every minute of every night exposes them to danger.

Sleep.

In this book, you will learn about sleep and how to improve it. You will learn why "sleep saves lives." You will learn that doing little things can make big changes. You will learn how to tell if you are getting the right amount and quality of sleep you need and what to do if you aren't. This book will give you the tools you need to improve your sleep.

Sleep.

The goal is that you go to bed, shut your eyes, and drift off, and then wake up alert and in a great mood, ready to conquer your day.

FOREWORD

TWO VERY FREQUENTLY ASKED QUESTIONS ARE: Is sleep necessary? And, how much sleep do I (we) need? We know the answers to these questions about sleep, and much, much more. The answer to the first question is that we cannot do without sleep. The tendency for a person to fall asleep increases steadily as wakefulness continues. There comes a point when it will not be possible to stay awake unless heroic methods are applied. We also know how to answer the second question for any individual. As a matter of fact, sleep professionals have accumulated and applied an encyclopedia of sleep-related knowledge. The problem, which we hope this book will play a role in solving, is that the knowledge about sleep is not being effectively transmitted to the public.

As with every other normal function of the human body, sleep has a panoply of abnormalities. There are over eighty specific sleep disorders, ranging from mild insomnia to potentially lethal stoppage of breathing when one falls asleep. Approximately 50 million people have one or more of these numerous sleep disorders. Some of the greatest problems in our society come from universal chronic sleep deprivation with its negative consequences, from minimal impaired performance all the way to catastrophic error. There are individuals in our society who are at death's door because of an undetected sleep disorder—usually obstructive sleep apnea—and there are those who are walking time bombs, such as sleep deprived bus drivers, pilots, and so on.

On the other hand, there is the as yet unexploited potential of enormous improvement in productivity and performance in just about everything, if there could be widespread elimination of chronic sleep loss and widespread detection and treatment of sleep disorders. It is quite likely that the actual cost of sleep deprivation and disorders has never been fully gauged. President Bill Clinton once said, "The only time I made mistakes was when I was tired." Imagine how productive our society would be if everyone got the proper amount of sleep! In the following pages you will find information, quizzes, and questionnaires that will help you recognize if you are sleep deprived or have a disorder, and if so what you can do about it. Sleep is a fundamental human need, so why not learn to maximize its benefits?

—William C. Dement, MD, PhD
Professor of Psychiatry and Behavioral Sciences,
Stanford University

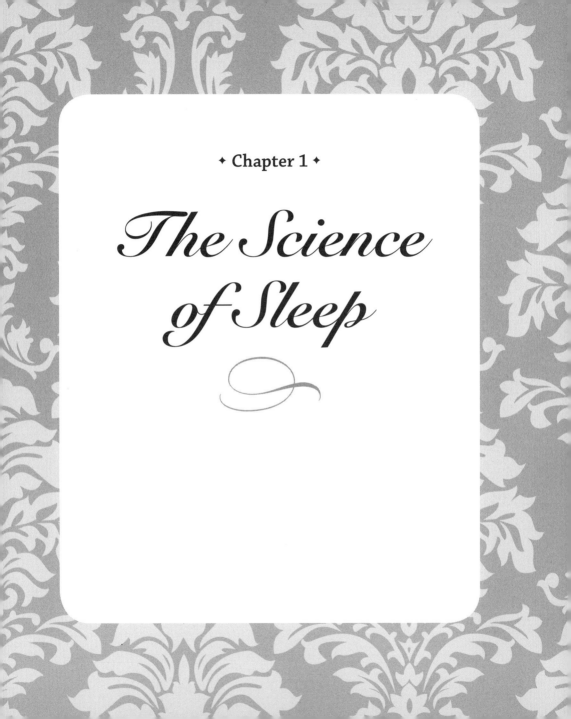

◆ Chapter 1 ◆

The Science of Sleep

ALL FORMS OF LIFE, from viruses to humans, have times when they are active and times when they are not. When organisms are not active, and if they have a nervous system, they exhibit what we call sleep. It is now known that these times of inactivity appear at regular intervals, almost as though controlled by a clock. It turns out that even organisms without a well-developed nervous system, such as insects, do, in fact, sleep. A hundred years ago, many people, including scientists, believed that sleep was a form of reversible death. In the last century, there emerged the notion that sleep was a type of hibernation state in which not much was happening. We now know that sleep is a very active state for our brains. During sleep, the brain is busy controlling breathing, heartbeat, and many other critical body functions, including the secretion of hormones. Also, it is now believed that during sleep a great deal of learning occurs and memories are stored on the hard drives of our brains.

WHY DO WE SLEEP?

There is no simple answer to the question of why we sleep, just as there is no simple answer to the question of why are we awake. A famous sleep scientist, Dr. Alan Rechtshaffen, once said that if sleep has no purpose, it is the biggest mistake evolution ever made. Many theories have evolved about why we sleep. What we do know is that sleep is a necessary function to live. Animals prevented from sleeping eventually die in what appears to be a horrible death. They become severely underweight, lose mental and physical abilities, and their fur falls out. A great deal of research has found that sleep is important for handling stress, promoting a strong immune system, and having the physical vitality and mental vigor to work, play, and eat. Good sleep also promotes a healthy heart and certainly contributes to a positive mood and good mental health. We can all easily recognize the moody, irritable person who has had a poor night's sleep.

WHEN DO WE SLEEP?

We generally go to bed at the same time every day and wake up at the same time every day. We even eat most of our meals at roughly the same time every day. Why do we establish these patterns? It turns out that almost all life forms have a natural internal clock system. Almost all organisms seem to do things at certain times of the day and night—this is even true for plants, some of which anticipate the position of the sun. Not only do people have a clock within them, but almost all the cells in the body also possess clocklike functions. In fact, over a twenty-four-hour period the functions of certain cells may change depending on the time of day or night. For example, in the middle of the night, when you are sleeping, you rarely need to go to the bathroom and do not become hungry. This is not just a coincidence. Scientists do not yet understand the entire internal body clock system, but there are some amazing clues and we have learned an enormous amount in just the past fifty years.

First, we have learned the location of the "master" clock in the body. This is a group of cells deep in the brain called the suprachiasmatic nucleus. These cells possess a clock function, almost like a pacemaker, and they communicate with all the other cells in the body. These cells are involved in the mechanism that produces melatonin, the natural hormone of darkness, which plays a role in sleep and wake regulation. This master body clock also controls our circadian rhythm. The circadian rhythm refers to the twenty-four-hour cycle of many of the body's functions. For example, body temperature has a twenty-four-hour cycle, rising with the sun in the morning and dropping at night when the lights go out.

HOW DOES THE MASTER BODY CLOCK KNOW WHAT TIME IT IS?

It turns out that what synchronizes the body clock in humans is light. Light stimulates receptors in the eye, which send impulses to the master body clock. Thus, every day your body clock synchronizes with the world. That is, it *would* synchronize with the world if sunlight were our only source of light. Artificial light sources have been trying to trick our brains into thinking it is time to be awake since the invention of the electric lamp. This is why you turn out the lights when you want to go to sleep.

> The circadian rhythm refers to the twenty-four-hour cycle of many of the body's functions.

WHAT CONTROLS WHEN WE SLEEP?

There are actually two factors that control when we sleep. The first is the master body clock, which signals the brain that it is time to sleep by shutting down an arousing effect. The other factor, not surprisingly, is how long we are awake. The longer we are awake, the sleepier we become. After about sixteen hours of being awake, most of us become sleepy. When that coincides with the master body clock reducing its arousing effect on the brain, a complex system takes over and we sleep.

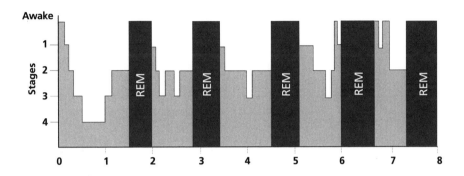

THE STAGES OF SLEEP

Whereas scientists once believed that sleep was a uniform state, they now know that it is much more complex. Sleep has been divided into stages that are easily identifiable in a laboratory. In humans there are four stages of non-dreaming sleep, and a separate stage of dreaming sleep.

Dreaming sleep is also called rapid eye movement, or REM sleep. The reason for this is that when we dream, there are rapid movements of our eyes. However, the rest of the body is usually in a state of paralysis—except for vital functions such as breathing and heartbeat.

In humans there are four stages of non-dreaming sleep, and a separate stage of dreaming sleep.

NON-REM SLEEP

Non-REM sleep is divided into four stages that are simply called 1, 2, 3, and 4. Stage 1 is when sleep is extremely light, and is often present when we first go to sleep and then only for a short period of time. It also occurs at other times during the night when we transition from one state to another. Stage 1 sleep usually makes up about 5 percent of total sleep time. Stage 2 sleep makes up about one half of the night, and stages 3 and 4 make up what is called slow wave sleep, which makes up about a quarter of the night in adults and much more in children. This stage is what scientists call the deepest stage of sleep. It is very difficult to awaken a person from slow wave sleep, and sometimes if you do, they might remain sleepy or confused. It is believed that this stage is the most important for growth and repair in our bodies.

> → In 1953, Dr. Nathaniel Kleitman, the "Father of American Sleep Research," and his student Eugene Aserinsky discovered the phenomenon of REM sleep. Shortly thereafter, in 1958, Dr. William C. Dement established the relationship between REM sleep and dreaming.

REM SLEEP

Rapid eye movement sleep is a wondrous state. It is the time when we have wonderful dreams and terrifying nightmares, but it is also a time when our bodies are almost entirely paralyzed, perhaps to prevent us from reacting to the content of our dreams.

BODY FUNCTIONS DURING SLEEP

In non-REM sleep, the body controls most of its functions very accurately. There is very little variability in heart rate, blood pressure, or breathing. On the other hand, during REM sleep it is almost as if the brain does not care about these normal functions, and they may become erratic. For example, the body stops controlling temperature. Another little-understood event that happens during REM sleep is that males will have erections of their penises, and females will have engorgement of their vaginal tissues. We have no clue why this might occur. It is not believed that these events are responses to sexual dreams or thoughts, because they actually can be documented shortly after birth.

HOW MUCH SLEEP DO WE NEED?

There are several ways to answer the question of how much sleep we need. The easiest and perhaps ultimately the most accurate answer is: the amount of sleep that leaves us feeling wide-awake, alert, and in a positive mood in the morning. There is no one answer for everybody. If you think about it, you probably already know how much sleep you need to achieve this state of feeling rested. However, there are different sleep needs during different stages of life. For example, children and adolescents require more sleep than adults. The table below tells you how much sleep is needed on average for people of different ages. The average adult needs seven to nine hours. It is very important to get the sleep you need; research shows that people who continuously sleep much less than seven hours or much more than nine hours have a higher death rate.

HOW MUCH SLEEP DO YOU REALLY NEED?	
AGE	**SLEEP NEEDS**
Newborns (1–2 months)	10.5–18 hours
Infants (3–11 months)	9–12 hours at night and 30-minute–2-hour naps, 1–4 times per day
Toddlers (1–3 years)	12–14 hours
Preschoolers (3–5 years)	11–13 hours
Children (5–12 years)	10–11 hours
Teens (13–17 years)	8.5–9.25 hours
Adults	7–9 hours
Older Adults	7–9 hours

As important as the number of hours of sleep is the quality of sleep. Sleep can be interrupted by anything from medical conditions that cause pain to a bed partner's snoring to taking care of children at night. When sleep is interrupted, even though a person may feel that they slept for the right number of hours, they may still suffer from daytime sleepiness or moodiness and an impaired ability to function mentally.

The irony is that some people who have serious disorders such as sleep apnea (which is described in Chapter Three) might think they are champion sleepers, but because of the sleep apnea their brains will frequently awaken more than once every minute during the night. It is these many unconscious awakenings that can result in severe sleepiness during the day.

We have all heard about famous people, sometimes billionaires, accomplished scientists, or inspiring artists, who claim that they only sleep three or four hours a night, because they believe that sleep is a waste of time and keeps them from their main purpose in life. Do not believe everything you hear. Although there are some people who can probably function well on four to six hours of sleep per night, at least for a short period of time, the vast majority of adults need somewhere between seven and nine hours.

SLEEP CAN SAVE YOUR LIFE!

Sleep saves lives in many ways. Without any sleep at all we would eventually die, like the animals mentioned earlier. But just getting enough sleep to live is not adequate either; we need the right amount of sleep to be healthy and productive and even just to feel good. Without sleep, none of us would be able to function in the way that we need to in order to do our jobs and take care of our families and ourselves.

Besides the fact that normal sleep is essential to your overall health, there are many other ways that sleep is critical. Without adequate sleep, people have fallen asleep while piloting aircraft and ships, driving trucks and automobiles, and operating heavy machinery—often with disastrous results. Rumble strips have been added to most of the nation's new highways to awaken people who have drifted off the road and are about to crash their vehicles. However, thousands of fall-asleep crashes occur every year on America's highways, resulting in thousands of needless deaths.

Without sleep, none of us would be able to function in the way that we need to in order to do our jobs and take care of our families and ourselves.

WHAT CAN BE WRONG WITH MY SLEEPING?

In this book we will cover many of the problems that can derail the normal sleep-wake cycle. In some people, the master body clock is abnormal and they may become sleepy much earlier or much later than the usual rhythm that most of us follow. For some, their brains are "overexcited" and they cannot fall asleep or stay asleep throughout the night. This leads to insomnia. Some people develop diseases like narcolepsy that result in their sleeping too much. And then there are those people who have diseases that continuously disrupt their sleep, leaving them feeling tired and unrefreshed in the morning. Such individuals may be in great danger. For example, with obstructive sleep apnea, patients stop breathing briefly during sleep, and this can have catastrophic outcomes on their health. Sometimes, sleep is affected by our lifestyle and the choices we make. Such sleep problems can also have catastrophic effects; for example, a sleep-deprived driver falling asleep at the wheel.

In this book you will learn how to assess your sleep and find out what to do if you have a sleep disorder.

◆ Chapter 2 ◆

Assessing Your

SLEEP DISORDER

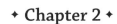

"WHAT SLEEP DISORDER? I sleep fine. In fact, I can fall asleep anywhere anytime." As a sleep professional, I can't tell you how often I have heard that line or a similar one. The truth is that a large percentage of people with sleep problems don't think they have one. I encounter two distinct groups all the time. The first are typified by feeling the way I stated above—people who are sleepier than they should be but don't realize it. The other group is those who have difficulty sleeping but think that is normal and they just have to live with it.

ARE YOU SLEEP DEPRIVED?

"How can I not realize I am sleepy?" you ask. It's easy; we as a society have gotten used to being sleepy. The first thing to realize is that after sleeping at night you should awaken refreshed and ready to go. If you need an alarm clock to wake you at your regular wake time, something is wrong! It's no more normal to wake up feeling groggy and slow to get going than it is to finish a full dinner and still feel hungry. Are you one of those people who reports that you sleep great, but you fall asleep almost as soon as your head hits the pillow? Do you think this is a good thing? It's not! If you are getting an adequate amount of good quality sleep, it will usually take you ten or fifteen minutes to fall asleep. If you fall asleep instantly there is a good chance that you are sleep deprived, whether from inadequate hours of sleep, poor quality of sleep, or both. As will soon become clearer, falling asleep instantly or sleeping anywhere anytime are not things to take pride in, they should raise a red flag that you may have a sleep problem.

If you need an alarm clock to wake you at your regular wake time, something is wrong!

Do you sit down to read and feel you could nod off easily? How about while watching TV? In the theater or a meeting? Riding in a car? If you rated your chance of this happening as fairly high, you are sleepy—sleepier that you should be or need to be. In fact, clinicians, health care providers, and researchers ask these and a few other questions—eight questions to be precise—and use the "score" as a valid measure of sleepiness. Maybe you are someone who seems to function fairly well and don't realize that you are actually not at peak performance because of insufficient or poor quality sleep.

Take the Epworth Sleepiness Scale quiz on the following page to see if you are sleepy or not.

Epworth Sleepiness Scale

(designed by Dr. Murray Johns of Australia)
©M.W. Johns 1990-1997

To assess your sleepiness, answer the questions below with your first reaction, rating the chance of dozing in each of the eight situations from 0, or no chance, to 3, a high chance.

Sitting and Reading

0	No chance of dozing
1	Slight chance of dozing
2	Moderate chance of dozing
3	High chance of dozing

Watching TV

0	No chance of dozing
1	Slight chance of dozing
2	Moderate chance of dozing
3	High chance of dozing

Sitting inactive in a public place, such as a theater or meeting

0	No chance of dozing
1	Slight chance of dozing
2	Moderate chance of dozing
3	High chance of dozing

As a passenger in a car for an hour without a break

0	No chance of dozing
1	Slight chance of dozing
2	Moderate chance of dozing
3	High chance of dozing

Lying down to rest in the afternoon when circumstances permit

0   No chance of dozing
1   Slight chance of dozing
2   Moderate chance of dozing
3   High chance of dozing

Sitting and talking to someone

0   No chance of dozing
1   Slight chance of dozing
2   Moderate chance of dozing
3   High chance of dozing

Sitting quietly after a lunch without alcohol

0   No chance of dozing
1   Slight chance of dozing
2   Moderate chance of dozing
3   High chance of dozing

In a car, while stopped for a few minutes in traffic

0   No chance of dozing
1   Slight chance of dozing
2   Moderate chance of dozing
3   High chance of dozing

Now add up your points. If you scored less than 8 you are not sleepy! But, if you scored 8 to 11 you have mild sleepiness, 12 to 15 you have moderate sleepiness, 16 to 24 you have severe sleepiness. Surprised?

Even if you got a low score on the Epworth Sleepiness Scale, you should be aware that even this well-recognized test misses a lot, because sleepiness can be present with much subtler signs. Sleepiness affects our behavior, thinking, and physical performance before it translates into actually falling asleep. Do you:

+ Feel irritable?
+ Have trouble with concentration and memory?
+ Find you are making errors in your work that you aren't used to?
+ React to events slower than usual?
+ Frequently get jolted by the rumble strips on the side of the road while driving?
+ Yawn frequently and have heavy eyelids?

These are subtle yet clear warning signals that you are not well rested, even if you think you are and seem to be functioning in your daily activities. Studies have shown that sleep-deprived individuals who think they are fine, are not. Tests of their reaction time, memory, and clarity of thought all show them to be impaired, yet they often deny having a problem.

GETTING THE RIGHT AMOUNT OF SLEEP

So how do people, healthy people without a sleep disorder, get into such trouble with sleep deprivation? It's simple: we just don't sleep enough. We don't give ourselves a chance to sleep the amount our body and brain need. Every person seems to have a unique amount of sleep that is best for them. How much sleep is that? Over the years, population surveys and studies in controlled environments have indicated that adults really do need about seven to nine hours of sleep each night to feel refreshed and able to awaken without an alarm clock. In fact, if you sleep a little more than seven hours, some studies suggest you may be even better rested. Studies have been conducted where the participant is isolated from any external clues as to what time it is—whether it is night or day, what mealtime it is, etc. These studies support the natural sleep need to be about eight hours or slightly more. Interestingly, these studies also suggest that our natural clocks are not exactly set for a twenty-four-hour day but more like twenty-four and a quarter hours. This finding helps explain why most people find it easier to stay up a little later and fall asleep than to go to sleep early and fall asleep. How little is still enough? No one can answer that for everyone, but certainly getting at least seven hours of sleep seems important. And again, closer to eight hours works best for most adults.

Over the years, population surveys and studies in controlled environments have indicated that adults really do need about seven to nine hours of sleep each night to feel refreshed and able to awaken without an alarm clock.

"But," you may say, "I always get five or six hours and I am fine. I've been doing it for years. I have no problems during the day. What about me? I guess that makes me one of those people you hear about who just doesn't need much sleep. Didn't President Clinton get along with very little sleep? I'm the same!"

Well, it turns out that Clinton began to realize that lack of sleep might be an issue. He was quoted in an interview as saying that every significant mistake he had made was related to a decision he made while being sleep deprived. He also said he suspected that a large part of the reason that there is so much rancor and partisanship in Congress is because the members are sleep deprived. He went on to describe the tough schedule that congressmen and senators face.

Sleep deprivation seems to be a common issue. Many Americans, as well as many in other industrialized nations, convince themselves they are okay with inadequate sleep. But by and large they are just in a state of denial. True so-called "short sleepers" are few and far between. Those who convince themselves they are among that group are usually those with busy schedules who believe they can learn to manage with less sleep. Well, it is true you can learn to get by on less sleep, but that is very different from needing less sleep. And that lack of sleep almost always rears its head in some negative way. Maybe some drop off at work, causing errors to be made. Maybe some lose patience with a family member, lashing out for no real reason. Or, more gravely, someone may suffer a moment of inattention, what is referred to in medical terms as a micro-sleep. This may not matter much if you are sitting in front of the computer screen, but if you're driving at seventy miles an hour, it can be long enough to put you in a ditch or over an embankment.

Drowsy driving is such an under-recognized issue with such tragic consequences that the National Sleep Foundation now sponsors a Drowsy Driving Prevention Week™. The Web site, www.drowsydriving.org, is filled with poignant and tragic tales of people, too often very young people, who have suffered life-changing injuries or death as a direct consequence of drowsy driving leading to serious crashes. It is probable that many of these drivers were in denial about their drowsiness. Don't become a statistic!

SLEEP QUALITY

Okay fine, you're someone who actually tries to get eight hours of sleep, but you still awaken groggy, and when you take the Epworth quiz, lo and behold, you come out with a score indicating you are in fact sleepy during the day. What's going on now?

Well, in addition to an adequate amount or quantity of sleep, the other determinant of feeling fully rested is the quality of sleep. Poor-quality sleep is often a result of poor sleep habits or one of a broad number of sleep disorders. Sleep disorders will be discussed in more detail in the next chapter, but let us understand how poor sleep can result from some conditions.

First, there are conditions called primary sleep disorders. When a person reports that they are getting eight hours of sleep, or sometimes even more, and are still sleepy during the day, there is a very high likelihood that they have one of these conditions.

> Poor-quality sleep is often a result of poor sleep habits or one of a broad number of sleep disorders.

Perhaps most serious from the medical point of view is obstructive sleep apnea, usually tipped off by the presence of loud, disruptive snoring. This does not automatically mean that every person who snores has sleep apnea, but it should be considered.

Narcolepsy is an uncommon though not rare disorder marked by daytime "sleep attacks," as well as other characteristic symptoms. And we are now aware that some individuals suffer from difficulties with involuntary leg movements, both before they fall asleep, making sleep onset difficult, and after sleep onset, causing brief arousals due to leg kicking during the night. This condition, called Restless Legs Syndrome, leaves the patient sleep deprived.

Most common in terms of sheer numbers is insomnia. Calling insomnia a primary sleep disorder may not be exactly accurate. Doctors recognize that some people do have primary insomnia—difficulty falling or staying asleep with no specific independent cause identified. Many more have secondary or co-morbid insomnia. In National Sleep Foundation surveys over the years, the widespread prevalence of insomnia has become obvious:

- ✦ Depending on criteria, as many as 50 to 60 percent of adults experience insomnia some of the time in any given year
- ✦ As many as 10 to 15 percent of adults have chronic insomnia—insomnia lasting more than four weeks
- ✦ Women report more insomnia than men
- ✦ There is an increasing incidence of insomnia with age

THE THREE P'S

Many patients with difficulty sleeping start out not having any problem, but then something in their lives triggers the onset of sleep problems. The "Three P's," developed by Dr. Art Spielman, will help give us an approach to understanding and dealing with insomnia. Doctors often say that those who are at risk suffer from Predisposing factors. These may include certain personality traits, such as a tendency towards anxiety or depression, or even just a genetic tendency towards hyperarousal, a biological difficulty to shut down at bedtime. But many patients can cruise along with these "predisposers" kept in check until *wham!*, something happens to Precipitate the onset of insomnia. Precipitating factors include outside events and stressors in life, mostly negative but sometimes even excitement about something good can precipitate insomnia. Once insomnia gets going, the trick is to try to nip it in the bud. But many individuals who experience the onset of sleep problems develop poor coping mechanisms. These Perpetuating factors actually contribute to the continuation of their insomnia. Insomnia will be discussed in more detail in the next chapter, but in the end, recognizing what is going on and finding effective ways to prevent perpetuation will be key.

OTHER MEDICAL CONDITIONS AND SLEEP

Sometimes the precipitating event that disrupts sleep may actually be a separate medical condition. Many diseases are unfortunately associated with sleep disruption. A couple of examples include arthritis pain that makes sleep difficult or shortness of breath from lung or heart disease that keeps patients awake. In such scenarios, treating the underlying disease is of great importance, but in recent years we have increasingly come to realize that treatment of the sleep disorder will help the patient to better deal with the disease, sometimes actually reducing symptoms. This is true of acute illness, but especially crucial in chronic conditions where sleep and symptoms are long-term issues that always need to be thought about together.

Women face particular challenges in maintaining healthy sleep patterns throughout their lives. The various stages of a woman's hormonal evolution often create sleep challenges for them. Women face sleep issues related to menstruation, pregnancy, and menopause. There are often mood swings in association with these hormonally driven stages, but add to that sleep disruption and the combination can seriously impact the quality of life for women.

> ## Women face sleep issues related to menstruation, pregnancy, and menopause.

RECOGNIZING IF YOU HAVE A SLEEP PROBLEM

The assessment of these problems starts with being open to considering a sleep disorder as a possible factor in the quality of your life and health. Many tools are available to help you recognize that you might have a sleep problem. We have mentioned a simple quiz, the Epworth Sleepiness Scale, on page 30, as a measure of daytime sleepiness. If your sleep patterns are a concern and you're not sure what is going on, a Sleep Log or Sleep Diary can often offer clues. This involves keeping track of your sleep and wake patterns, including interruptions, for one to two weeks. Reviewing this log can point to a specific problem and greatly facilitate decisions as to what further studies, if any, are needed, or where to begin some form of treatment. Once you begin to home in on the presence of a sleep problem, you will be able to go to your primary healthcare provider and seek help.

Take the following quiz to help assess whether you have a sleep disorder and to help prepare you for the next chapter.

Sleep Disorder Assessment Quiz

Check if any of the following apply to you:

❑ Snoring loudly

❑ You or others have observed that you stop breathing or gasp for breath during sleep

❑ Feeling sleepy or dozing off while watching television, reading, driving, or engaged in daily activities

❑ Having difficulty sleeping three nights a week or more (e.g., trouble falling asleep, waking frequently during the night, or waking too early and unable to fall back asleep)

❑ Experiencing unpleasant, tingling, creeping feelings in your legs, or nervousness and the urge to move your legs when trying to sleep

❑ Experiencing interruptions to your sleep (e.g., nighttime heartburn, bad dreams, pain, discomfort, noise, sleep difficulties of family members, light, or temperature)

If you checked more than one box, you may be at risk of having a sleep disorder.

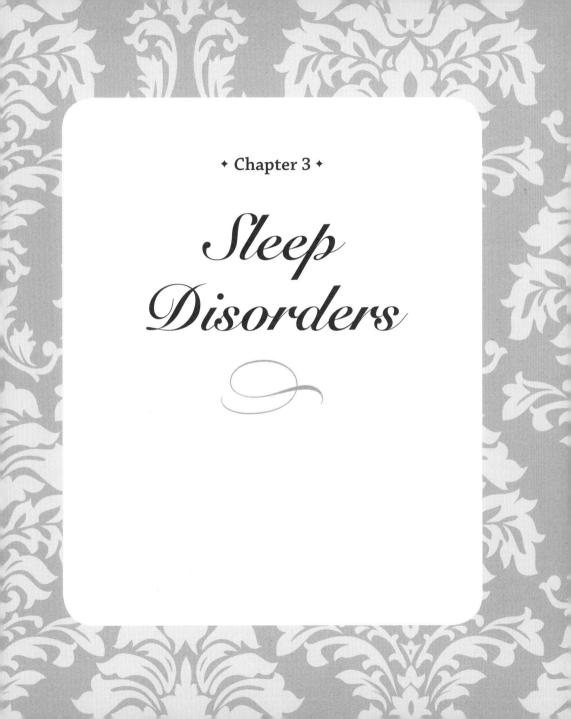

✦ Chapter 3 ✦

Sleep Disorders

SLEEP DISORDERS are a lot more common than you might think. According to the Institute of Medicine (IOM), 50 to 70 million Americans suffer from some chronic disorder of sleep and wakefulness. It's important to know that sleep disorders are serious medical conditions and have health consequences ranging from poor mental health to hypertension and even stroke. In this chapter, you will learn about some of the most common sleep disorders, how you might recognize them in yourself or your family, and what some of the options for treatment are that you could consider with your healthcare professional.

INSOMNIA

Everyone knows what insomnia is and if they have it, right?

Actually, it's not quite so clear what it is, who has it, and why, not to mention what to do about it if you do have it.

First of all, what do sleep specialists mean when they talk about insomnia? Insomnia is defined as difficulty falling asleep and staying asleep and/or waking up too early or feeling unrefreshed in the morning, resulting in daytime consequences. These daytime consequences might include problems with performing work, mood abnormalities such as irritability and impatience, and other problems related to daytime sleepiness.

It used to be thought that insomnia was always a symptom of some other disease, but we now know that this is not necessarily true. Insomnia is found as a symptom of many medical conditions, like depression, heart failure, and arthritis—

in fact, almost any medical condition—and sometimes the medications we use to treat those conditions can lead to insomnia. When insomnia is present along with another medical condition, they are referred to as being "co-morbid." This label actually represents an important shift in thinking about insomnia, and has resulted in a new approach to treatment. This shift is a result of a 2005 National Institutes of Health (NIH) "State of the Art" conference of experts. At an earlier conference in 1983, the theory was as stated above—that insomnia was always secondary to another underlying condition. It was felt that if the underlying condition was treated, then the insomnia would disappear, so there was no real need to focus on the insomnia itself. Temporary measures—usually intermittent use of sleeping pills—were considered adequate treatment. As a result of the 2005 conference, however, it was acknowledged that while insomnia can be related to a medical condition, it is its own condition as well, and often warrants aggressive treatment. Treating both the underlying medical ailment and the insomnia at the same time may lead to improved and more rapid results in both the condition and the insomnia.

Insomnia is defined as difficulty falling asleep and staying asleep and/or waking up too early or feeling unrefreshed in the morning, resulting in daytime consequences.

BUT WHY DO SOME PEOPLE HAVE PROBLEMS AND NOT OTHERS?

As we discussed in Chapter Two, some people are more "Predisposed" to developing difficulties with sleep. They may have a chronic disease caused by a hyperaroused state of the nervous system manifesting itself in difficulty falling asleep and staying asleep. In fact, some people who have insomnia have no other medical or psychiatric conditions whatsoever, and in many of them, it turns out that the problem has been present for many years, often since birth. Insomnia may also run in families. This is called primary insomnia.

Some individuals don't develop insomnia until a stressful situation or other life event occurs. This is the "Precipitating" event; it can uncover a tendency for insomnia in someone who had previously never had a problem with sleep. This can leave a person frustrated and confused. What happened to me? Is it ever going to end? These individuals often develop poor behaviors and coping mechanisms that they use when they have insomnia. The things they try can actually "Perpetuate" the problem long after the stressful event has been resolved. Sometimes, people will have evidence of insomnia for years after the initial stressful event. For example, a new mother gets awakened frequently by her child. She begins to suffer from this recurring pattern of awakenings. Although her child eventually develops a more regular sleep pattern and begins to sleep through the night, some mothers continue to have a pattern of insomnia, with one or multiple awakenings per night, even when the precipitating event is gone.

HOW COMMON IS IT?

Insomnia is extremely common. It occurs in all age groups, but the percentage of the population that has it increases with age. Insomnia is found in probably 40 to 50 percent of older adults and 20 to 40 percent of younger adults. In all age groups, insomnia is more common in women than it is in men. Insomnia with negative daytime consequences is found in about 10 to 15 percent of the population.

It is important to emphasize that just because a person is older does not mean that he or she will have insomnia. Many older people, if they do not have any medical or psychiatric problems, may sleep just fine. The more medical and psychiatric conditions a person has, the more likely they are to have insomnia. Women may be more likely to experience insomnia because they are more likely to be diagnosed with depression, which insomnia is often associated with, and are much more likely to have their sleep interrupted because of changes in hormone levels during menstruation, pregnancy, and the peri and menopausal years.

> Insomnia is found in probably 40 to 50 percent of older adults and 20 to 40 percent of younger adults. In all age groups, insomnia is more common in women than it is in men.

DO I HAVE INSOMNIA?

Insomnia is defined as difficulty falling asleep and staying asleep and/or waking up too early and feeling unrefreshed in the morning, resulting in daytime sleepiness and its consequences. These consequences might include problems performing work, distress, and mood abnormalities.

There is a factor in the evaluation of insomnia that has always been puzzling to healthcare providers. You can have two people, both of whom will tell you it takes them twenty minutes to fall asleep at night. One will tell you that the twenty minutes is normal and not a problem, while the other will be very distressed by how long it takes her/him to fall asleep. When some people wake up at night they will simply fall asleep again in five minutes and do not see this as an issue, whereas others look at their alarm clocks, become distressed, and have difficulty falling back asleep.

You have insomnia if it takes you more than twenty minutes to fall asleep and/ or you wake up at night and cannot fall back to sleep for more than twenty minutes three or more nights a week for at least three months. This leads to distress, non-refreshing sleep, and mood changes that have a negative impact on your day.

HOW IS INSOMNIA TREATED?

First, since insomnia is often associated with other conditions, it is important that those other conditions be dealt with. For example, if a person has severe depression or stress, those conditions need to be treated. If the insomnia persists after treatment of other problems, then it will need to be specifically treated. Recently there has been a trend to treat insomnia earlier.

Second, review your sleep habits (see Chapter Eight). Make sure that your sleep environment (bedroom, etc.) is sleep promoting, that your internal environment is sleep promoting (relaxed, unstressed), and that you haven't done anything that would interfere with your ability to sleep, for example working late into the night, using your computer or watching television right before bed, or balancing your checkbook. If you have not already done so, develop sleep-promoting habits like a warm bath or a nighttime ritual, which can be very helpful.

You might also try some cognitive behavioral exercises. Sleep habits and cognitive behavioral exercises are reviewed in Chapter Eight.

WHEN TO SEEK PROFESSIONAL HELP

If your insomnia distresses you and you have not been able to cure it yourself, then you should seek professional help. Interestingly, only a small percentage of individuals with insomnia bring it up to their healthcare providers, and healthcare providers frequently fail to ask about their patients' sleep. With the advent of direct-to-consumer marketing of newer sleeping pills, there does seem to be an increase in patients recognizing that there are things that can be done for insomnia.

> Although sleeping pills may end up being a solution for you, you deserve a lot more than a five-minute doctor visit and a sleeping pill prescription.

Although sleeping pills may end up being a solution for you, you deserve a lot more than a five-minute doctor visit and a sleeping pill prescription. Prescribing sleeping pills is not the first or only treatment that should be considered when insomnia is present. Your practitioner should always discuss the problems that may be causing your insomnia, behaviors that you have that might be perpetuating the insomnia, and sleep habits before deciding whether you need additional help from medications or a sleep specialist or clinical psychologist.

The National Sleep Foundation has a program on its Web site at www.sleepfoundation.org that will help you understand what to expect from cognitive behavioral treatment provided by a psychologist.

THE GOOD NEWS!

The good news is that in most cases, insomnia can be treated successfully and you will no longer feel distressed at the thought of not sleeping. You will not be afraid to go to sleep.

SNORING

Snoring is a breathing sound made during sleep that occurs when the upper breathing passage is obstructed. It is caused by vibration in the tissues of the upper breathing passage. The noise from snoring can range from a soft purring noise to almost as loud as a jackhammer if it occurs next to a bed partner's ear. Most of the time snoring is not dangerous, but it can be quite a challenge for a bed partner—and often other family members in the house—to sleep through. Snoring is a common symptom of sleep apnea, which is discussed in the next section, but most people who snore do not have sleep apnea.

DO I SNORE?

Unless someone has told you that you snore, you probably don't know whether you do or not. Clues that snoring is present include awakening every morning with a sore or dry throat and sometimes with a swollen uvula (that little thing that hangs down at the back of your throat). You may also have unexplained high blood pressure. If you find that you awaken frequently with your bed partner sleeping in another room or if a neighbor banging on the wall awakens you at night, you should be suspicious. Risk factors that can cause snoring include:

- Being overweight
- Having a small jaw or a significant overbite
- Nasal congestion, whether due to a cold or allergies or chronic inflammation
- Nasal obstruction such as with a deviated septum
- Sleeping with your mouth open
- Getting older

It used to be thought that women rarely snore, but it is now clear that women snore almost as often as men do. It is just not discussed as often.

IS SNORING DANGEROUS?

Snoring by itself is not dangerous, but it may be a symptom of something more serious. Snoring causes sleep difficulties for bed partners, and may lead to relationship problems. Often a spouse will choose to sleep in another room, putting a strain on the relationship. The divorce rate has been reported as being higher with a snorer in the family. Snoring may curtail travel since the couple can't imagine sleeping in the same room. Sometimes the snoring is so disruptive of other people's sleep that violence has been committed in an attempt to stop the racket.

DO I NEED TO SEE MY DOCTOR IF I SNORE?

If you have no other symptoms of sleep apnea (see page 53) and do not have any indication of cardiovascular disease, then probably not. Sometimes people need help for snoring because it has caused problems with relationships with bed partners and friends.

Often the bed partner will initially try to fall asleep first, but that doesn't always work. Next they will try earplugs. Finally they will sleep elsewhere. Encouraging the snorer to go to the doctor for evaluation is often the next step.

WHAT CAN BE DONE ABOUT SNORING?

Avoid alcohol

Alcohol is known to make snoring worse and should be avoided after supper.

Lose weight

Some people only snore when overweight.

An oral appliance

Consider speaking to your dentist about using an oral appliance. Certain oral appliances, which bring the lower jaw up and forward, are often very effective in reducing snoring.

Sleep on your side

Sleeping on the side will often help snorers, especially those who sleep with their mouths wide open. This is unfortunately sometimes difficult to achieve consistently.

Nasal strips

In some cases, snoring is caused by an obstruction in the nasal breathing passages. Nasal strips, which spread apart the opening of the nose, are effective in some snorers but not all.

Controversial treatments: surgery and anti-snoring gadgets

In general, surgical procedures that deal with snoring may be only partially effective, or completely ineffective, and it depends on your anatomy. All sorts of gimmicky surgical procedures have been introduced, but many such operations are not recommended because they have not been scientifically shown to be consistently effective.

There are many gadgets, including sprays, pillows, and beds, that have been introduced with the claim that they treat snoring. By and large, these products, often marketed in magazines, on television, or on the Internet, are not particularly effective for most people and thus are not recommended. For example, I would not recommend that someone spend $200 on a pillow to treat snoring since such pillows have not been shown scientifically to work for most people.

SLEEP APNEA

The word apnea means "not breathing." Sleep apnea is a condition in which people stop breathing during sleep. In most cases of sleep apnea, a person may stop breathing anywhere from five to sixty or more times each hour. Every time one stops breathing, in order to start again the brain temporarily wakes up to initiate breathing. In some cases, it is so severe that a person literally cannot breathe and sleep at the same time.

There are two types of sleep apnea. The more common is called obstructive sleep apnea. In this type, as the person struggles to breathe in, the upper breathing passage literally collapses. We are not aware of the muscles working to help us breathe. Even when we are awake, we don't think about breathing. What we don't realize is that in addition to the chest expanding to draw air in, there are muscles in the throat, or pharynx, that also participate in breathing. The pharynx has no rigid structure to hold it open while taking a breath. Without being aware of it, the muscles in the pharynx actively hold the throat open, allowing air to enter our lungs. In obstructive sleep apnea, when the patient falls asleep something about going to sleep causes a loss of muscle tone in the pharynx that allows it to collapse and obstruct air flow. The brain is able to recognize that the person is literally choking and briefly awakens him or her from sleep, allowing the muscles to work and open the airway again. Patients with obstructive sleep apnea are therefore often observed to stop breathing for a period of time, ranging from ten seconds to more than sixty seconds. This "apnea" is terminated with a gasp or snort, often even louder than snoring.

> → **Obstructive sleep apnea was first described not by a clinical doctor, but by Charles Dickens, in 1836. In his book *The Pickwick Club*, Dickens depicted an excessively sleepy, overweight boy named Joe who snored and may have had right-sided heart failure. For many years, obstructive sleep apnea was called the "Pickwickian syndrome." However, obstructive sleep apnea was not recognized as a clinical disorder until more than a hundred and twenty years after Dickens' description.**

Patients themselves are almost never aware of the events just mentioned and are shocked to find out they have been waking up, even if only for a few seconds, many times a night—sometimes even hundreds of times a night. Occasionally, patients are aware of something waking them but don't know what it is. They often think they are waking to go to the bathroom, but when their apnea is finally treated, the need to urinate at night often disappears. Some patients do realize that they occasionally wake up gasping and choking. Some will actually report that they frequently dream they are drowning or suffocating. But overall, they have little idea of what is going on as they sleep.

The second type of apnea is called central sleep apnea. In this type, more often found in people with heart failure or those who have a nervous system problem, patients simply stop trying to breathe, over and over during the night. We will focus on the much more common obstructive sleep apnea in this section.

HOW COMMON IS IT?

Sleep apnea is an extremely common condition that is found in all age groups from newborns to people in their nineties. Most people go to the doctor when symptoms are severe or when there is concern expressed by a bed partner, most often when they are in their forties. Sleep apnea is found in at least 2 percent of women and 4 percent of men. More recent data suggest that the figure is probably higher than that.

HOW DO I KNOW IF I HAVE SLEEP APNEA?

The main symptoms of sleep apnea are related to severe daytime sleepiness that result from repeated awakenings during the night. People have problems with their memory and their ability to concentrate, or they may fall asleep when they do not want to, including during meetings or while operating a motor vehicle. Many patients initially think they have insomnia, as they don't realize what is keeping them from sleeping well. In fact, it is not unusual to find patients with sleep apnea who have been treated with sleeping pills. It is important to point out that women with sleep apnea are much more likely to have insomnia as a clinical symptom.

You may have sleep apnea if:

+ You have an Epworth Sleepiness Scale score of more than 10 (take the quiz on page 30)

+ You sleep seven to eight hours but still feel unrefreshed in the morning and don't really feel good until after a shower or a cup of coffee, or you never feel refreshed at all.

+ You snore loudly and have been observed to stop breathing, gasp, or snort during sleep

+ You are overweight or have a neck size over seventeen inches in men or sixteen inches in women

+ You have a body mass index (BMI) of 30 or more and are considered obese. A tool to calculate your BMI is at www.nhlbisupport.com/bmi.

+ You awaken with a dry mouth and often with a headache

+ You have trouble concentrating and your memory isn't as sharp as it used to be

+ You have a small jaw, enlarged tonsils, or nasal obstruction

+ You go to the bathroom several times at night but have no history of diabetes or urinary tract problems or, if you are a man, enlarged prostate

+ Others in your family have had sleep apnea—there is a strong genetic component

A diagnosis of sleep apnea is often missed because of stereotypes. For example, we used to think that it was only obese patients who had sleep apnea. While weight is a factor in a high percentage of sleep apnea cases, it has become clear that even slim people can have it.

Take the Berlin Questionnaire on the following page to help you determine if you might have sleep apnea.

Modified Berlin Questionnaire

Answer the following questions to the best of your ability.

CATEGORY 1: Snoring

1) Do you snore?

Yes   No   *Don't know*

If you answered yes:

2) Your snoring is:

a. Louder than talking

b. As loud as talking

c. Slightly louder than breathing

3) How often do you snore?

a. Nearly every night

b. 3 to 4 times a week

c. 1 to 2 times a week

d. 1 to 2 times a month

e. Never or almost never

4) Has your snoring ever bothered other people?

Yes   No

5) According to your own experiences or what others have told you, how often have you stopped breathing while sleeping?

a. Nearly every night

b. 3 to 4 times a week

c. 1 to 2 times a week

d. 1 to 2 times a month

e. Never or almost never

If you answered "Yes" or "a" or "b" to more than two questions, this category is positive.

CATEGORY 2: Sleeping

6) How often do you feel tired or fatigued immediately after waking up?

    a. Nearly every day

    b. 3 to 4 times a week

    c. 1 to 2 times a week

    d. 1 to 2 times a month

    e. Never or almost never

7) During the daytime, how often do you feel tired, fatigued, or not up to par?

    a. Nearly every day

    b. 3 to 4 times a week

    c. 1 to 2 times a week

    d. 1 to 2 times a month

    e. Never or almost never

8) Have you ever nodded off or fallen asleep while driving a vehicle?

    Yes   No

9) If you answered "Yes" to the last question, how often does this occur?

    a. Nearly every day

    b. 3 to 4 times a week

    c. 1 to 2 times a week

    d. 1 to 2 times a month

    e. Never or almost never

If you answered "Yes" or "a" or "b" to more than two questions, this category is positive.

CATEGORY 3: Risk Factors

10) Do you have high blood pressure?

    Yes   No   Don't know

11) Is your BMI (Body Mass Index) more than 30 or is your neck collar size bigger than 17 inches?

    Yes   No   Don't know

12) Do you have a very small jaw or a large overbite?

    Yes   No   Don't know

If you answered "Yes" to more than two questions, this category is positive.

To calculate your risk of apnea, check each category as positive or negative

  1. Snoring Category

      ❏ Positive   ❏ Negative

  2. Sleepiness Category

      ❏ Positive   ❏ Negative

  3. Risk Factors Category

      ❏ Positive   ❏ Negative

If two or more categories are positive, the chance that apnea is present is high.

Table 2 from Netzer NC, et al. Using the Berlin Questionnaire To Identify Patients at Risk for the Sleep Apnea Syndrome. *Ann Intern Med.* 1999; 131: 485–491.

The previous questionnaire indicates the likelihood that a person has sleep apnea. Some people who score positive might turn out not to have sleep apnea, while some who score negative might turn out to have it. To receive an accurate diagnosis of sleep apnea, the best course is to participate in an overnight sleep-study with polysomnography.

WHAT ARE THE RISKS OF SLEEP APNEA?

When someone stops breathing, their blood oxygen level drops, stress hormones and hormones that normally increase only during exercise are released, blood pressure goes up, and heart rate decreases then increases. These all have an effect of putting the individual at increased risk for health problems. Many people with sleep apnea have high blood pressure and may develop heart disease.

I THINK I HAVE SLEEP APNEA, WHAT NOW?

If you have some of the signs of sleep apnea—even if you don't have all of them—start by discussing the symptoms with your doctor. Most people at high risk for sleep apnea can expect to be referred to a sleep specialist and/or have an overnight sleep test to confirm the diagnosis. This test is called a polysomnogram. It involves going to a sleep laboratory and spending the night. During the night, sleep technicians measure multiple physiologic parameters, including your brain waves, to see how much you sleep and how many times you awaken. They will also observe your breathing, heart rate, muscle tone, and movement. There is no pain or discomfort associated with this, though it can certainly feel a little odd sleeping in a strange room with wires all over you and a sleep technician watching you all night.

Many people with sleep apnea have high blood pressure and may develop heart disease.

Once the diagnosis of sleep apnea is confirmed, most of the time the patient will have an additional sleep study to determine the best treatment for them, which often is continuous positive airway pressure, usually called CPAP.

CPAP

CPAP is a prescribed medical device made up of a mask that fits over the nose and/or mouth attached to a blower that generates pressure. Remember, in obstructive sleep apnea, the muscles in the pharynx lose their tone, allowing the airway to collapse. This pressure enlarges the opening in the upper breathing passage and keeps it from collapsing shut. The pressure level is usually determined during the sleep study, and patients are sent home with a machine that they usually will have to use as long as their main apnea risk factor (such as obesity) is present. When the possibility of wearing a mask is first mentioned, many patients' initial reaction is to completely reject the idea. In fact, some patients will actually refuse to go for the sleep study, stating that they are just not going to wear "that thing" no matter what. This is unfortunate, because in the majority of patients, with proper fitting and training in its use, CPAP can be life changing. Patients with daytime symptoms often feel they have been given a new lease on life. Many who were initially skeptical find it hard if not almost impossible to sleep without CPAP.

Today, there are many different masks and variations on the basic machine, which have made CPAP much more comfortable and tolerable for patients.

Dental or oral devices

Some patients do very well with a prescribed device to wear at night that brings the lower jaw up and forward. These devices have been approved for the treatment of mild to moderate sleep apnea but they are not usually effective when there is severe obesity or sleep apnea. Some patients will actually have both an oral appliance and CPAP. If you plan to ask your dentist about an oral appliance, make sure he or she has experience in such treatment. Don't be embarrassed to ask.

Avoid alcohol and sleeping pills

Patients with sleep apnea generally do better if they avoid alcohol, since alcohol has an effect of reducing the tone of the muscles that keep the breathing passage open during sleep. Patients should also avoid medications that have similar effects, such as some sleeping pills.

Losing weight

Losing weight can have an extremely beneficial effect on apnea. In fact, it is one of the only ways to possibly cure sleep apnea. Sleep apnea is present in a very high percentage of patients with morbid obesity. With the advent of bariatric surgery (intestinal bypass surgery), the massive weight loss that occurs with success of this treatment often resolves the patient's sleep apnea. Normalizing weight should always be one of the main goals of treatment.

THE GOOD NEWS!

Most patients do very well with treatment of their sleep apnea and their symptoms most often resolve.

RESTLESS LEGS SYNDROME

Restless legs syndrome (RLS) is one of those diseases that has a strange name and sounds like someone just made it up. In fact it is a common problem, first described hundreds of years ago, and is a condition in which patients have extremely unpleasant sensations in their legs and sometimes arms that keep them from falling asleep. This disorder is genetic in many patients, but in some patients it can be caused by a deficiency of iron, B12, or folic acid.

> → **RLS has often been considered a "made up" disease and was not taken very seriously by the public and medical community until July 2007, when researchers discovered genes linked to RLS and Periodic Limb Movement, establishing credibility for the very existence of the disease.**

HOW COMMON IS IT?

RLS is found in about 10 to 15 percent of the adult population, and in about 30 to 40 percent of the older population. It can even occur in children, but because they can have difficulty describing their symptoms they are sometimes misdiagnosed with ADHD, or even growing pains. It is much more common in people who have diabetes and kidney disease. Sometimes it will start during pregnancy. People who have donated excessive amounts of blood are also at risk of developing RLS because they may become iron deficient.

DO I HAVE RESTLESS LEGS SYNDROME?

People use many words to describe the RLS sensations in their legs. Some people describe their legs as being hot. One patient described the symptoms as though someone were very lightly touching his skin with their fingertips continuously and in a very unpleasant way. Some patients say that it feels like insects crawling underneath their skin. Patients have trouble falling asleep, tossing and turning to try to get comfortable, and feel the urge to move their legs or get up and walk around. Some people become so dead tired that they just cannot drag themselves out of bed to do this. Others find that getting out of bed and walking makes them feel more comfortable. Some patients cool their legs and feet using water or wet towels, and some immerse their feet in water as hot as they can bear to calm the unpleasant sensation.

About 70 percent of people with restless legs syndrome have twitching in their legs about every twenty to forty seconds all night long. These twitches are easily recorded during a sleep study. Bed partners of patients who have restless legs syndrome will remark that the patient moves a great deal during sleep, or may demonstrate other activities such as kicking or twisting.

If you have experienced the sensations mentioned above and they are generally worse at night and are relieved by movement, then it is very likely that you have restless legs syndrome. In addition, many people with this syndrome are fidgety during the daytime, especially when they are supposed to sit still, for example, at a theater or on an airplane.

> About 70 percent of people with restless legs syndrome have twitching in their legs about every twenty to forty seconds all night long.

HOW IS RESTLESS LEGS SYNDROME TREATED?

First, go to your doctor. It is important to make sure that the syndrome is not being caused by a deficiency of iron, B12, or folic acid. This can be ruled out with a simple blood test. If none of these deficiencies are present and if the condition is severe, causing significant distress or insomnia, then it might be helpful to try some of the medications that have recently been approved by the FDA for restless legs syndrome.

These medications include Requip® and Mirapex®. Many patients are frightened by the fact that these medications are also used to treat Parkinson's disease. However, they also appear to be effective in treating RLS.

DOES THE DISEASE GET BETTER?

RLS usually responds well to treatment, but in most people it is a lifelong condition, unless one of the nutritional deficiencies mentioned above is found and treated.

NARCOLEPSY

People with narcolepsy have severe sleepiness that often begins during the teenage years, and is frequently not noticed or diagnosed by the patient or the physician. Often it takes ten or more years before a definitive diagnosis is made, even though the patient has classic symptoms. Narcolepsy seems to run in families.

In narcolepsy, what normally only happens during rapid eye movement (REM) sleep occurs at the wrong time and place. The main cause of narcolepsy is thought to be a deficiency of specific transmitters in the central nervous system.

HOW COMMON IS NARCOLEPSY?

It used to be thought that narcolepsy was a rare condition, affecting perhaps one in two thousand people. It is now believed to be more common.

HOW DO I KNOW IF I HAVE NARCOLEPSY?

REM sleep is when we do most of our dreaming. During REM, presumably to keep us from acting out our dreams, our muscles are "paralyzed." With narcolepsy, the patient can have any of the parts of REM occur suddenly when he or she is wide awake. The most common complaint is of severe daytime sleepiness resulting in falling asleep, sometimes rather suddenly, at the wrong time or in the wrong place. Think of how this looks in school or on the job if no one, including the patient, knows what is causing such behavior.

> → **It wasn't until 1999 that Dr. Emmanuel Mignot and his team of researchers at Stanford University discovered the gene that causes narcolepsy.**

Another symptom that is present in many patients is very vivid dream imagery when they first fall asleep or when they wake up. This dream imagery can occur even before they are sound asleep. Other symptoms include sudden loss of muscle tone during the daytime, often in response to emotions or laughter. Sometimes the patient will collapse to the ground, and other times only a few muscle groups will be affected—for example, the facial muscles. A person does not lose consciousness with these episodes. As you can imagine, this can be frightening or embarrassing. Since this is a condition that often starts in the teenage years, think of a teenager who is asked to give a speech in class. The anxiety associated with this can trigger cataplexy, the medical name for sudden weakness, so he or she has to sit down and may not be able to function. Or, an excited teen hits a home run, and the excitement triggers an episode and he or she falls on the way to first base. Patients with narcolepsy can be mislabeled as lazy, strange, etc., until a diagnosis that explains these occurrences is made.

Sleep paralysis

Sometimes patients will awaken with paralysis of all their major muscle groups and they cannot move. This can be particularly frightening. Many people who experience such paralysis will also have the perception that there's someone else in the room as they are going to sleep or when they wake up in the middle of the night. This occasionally occurs in people without narcolepsy as well.

HOW IS NARCOLEPSY DIAGNOSED?

A diagnosis is confirmed by getting an overnight sleep observation that excludes other causes of severe daytime sleepiness, such as sleep apnea, followed by a daytime test called the Multiple Sleep Latency Test. In this test, the patient is given four or five opportunities to nap about every two hours during the daytime. The length of time it takes to fall asleep during these opportunities and whether or not they went into REM sleep are determined. Most patients with narcolepsy fall asleep in less than five minutes during the naps and they will have two or more episodes of REM sleep within their naps. People without narcolepsy will take much longer to fall asleep during the opportunities to nap and will not have REM sleep.

TREATMENT

There are medications currently available that deal with the symptoms of narcolepsy, since there is no known cure.

Medications that are used to make a person more alert during the daytime include Modafinil, Ritalin, and sometimes amphetamines. Other medications are used to treat other symptoms, like cataplexy. The most recent treatment approved that treats cataplexy as well as sleepiness is XYREM. Sometimes patients will be treated with drugs that are known to reduce REM sleep.

It is extremely important for a youngster who has narcolepsy to be accom-modated by the educational system. Specifically, patients with narcolepsy do extremely well after a brief nap. Some will have a nap shortly after lunch and another after returning home from school. Generally, patients will have a second wind for a couple of hours after such a nap.

REM SLEEP BEHAVIOR DISORDER

REM sleep behavior disorder is a condition in which patients appear to physically react to what they are dreaming. This used to be considered a very rare condition, but most sleep specialists have now seen many cases.

WHAT ARE THE SYMPTOMS?

When we are in REM or dreaming sleep, we are paralyzed. In patients with REM sleep behavior disorder, the mechanisms that cause paralysis in REM sleep do not function well, and when they dream they frequently react physically to the dream content. For example, if they have a dream that they are being attacked by a wolf, they may strike out and hurt themselves or their bed partner. Patients usually seek medical help precisely because one or both of those have happened. Although it is most commonly seen in older people, it sometimes can occur at a very young age. Recent research suggests that a significant proportion of people who have REM sleep behavior disorder will ultimately develop Parkinson's disease or a serious neurodegenerative disease in which major parts of the brain are affected.

TREATMENT

Patients with this disorder should be evaluated in a sleep clinic by a specialist and started on treatment. The most commonly used treatments include a drug called

Clonazepam that is effective in most cases. More recently, researchers have tried medications normally used for Parkinson's disease to see whether they can prevent the development of the more serious conditions that sometimes occur.

SLEEPWALKING, TALKING, SINGING, EATING, AND ALL THAT JAZZ

These conditions are called disorders of partial arousal. This means that parts of the brain are awake or aroused while others are still sound asleep. The part of the brain that deals with consciousness is asleep whereas the parts of the brain that control some muscle activity are functioning. People can do many strange things when they sleep. Some may cook, eat, wander around the house, or sing. In general, they have no recollection of having done these things.

HOW COMMON ARE THESE DISORDERS?

These disorders are extraordinarily common, and may affect 15 to 20 percent of children. They become less frequent as people become older. However, they still occur in adults and can be embarrassing.

HOW DO I KNOW IF I HAVE ONE OF THESE CONDITIONS?

Most of the time, people do not have any recollection of these types of behaviors during sleep. They become aware of them when someone tells them about it, or in the morning they find that something in the house is not exactly where it should be. Sometimes people will even eat in the middle of the night and have no recollection of it.

One type of partial arousal disorder, sleep terror, is particularly frightening to observers. The sleeper will appear to have awakened during the night and may scream, yell, and get up with sweat dripping from their foreheads with their eyes wide open, looking like they might commit a violent act. People are surprised to learn that this is a variant of sleepwalking, and that people have no recollection of these episodes unless told about them the next day, or if they are awakened during the episodes.

> → **Sleepwalking can be humorous but is often dangerous. I once had a patient who walked outside and was found wandering in a cemetery in the middle of the night in the dead of winter and had no recollection of it in the morning. Another patient, a businesswoman, often walked in her sleep when she traveled and stayed in hotels. One night she walked out of her room and got locked out in her pajamas.**
>
> **—Dr. Meir Kryger**

IS THERE TREATMENT FOR THESE CONDITIONS?

Yes, but first the factors increasing their likelihood need to be dealt with. The most common factor is sleep deprivation, and the second is the use of alcohol. Sleep deprivation is the easiest to deal with. When people finally realize that not getting enough sleep is leading to these often very embarrassing episodes, it is amazing how quickly most solve the problem by sleeping more. Similarly, reducing or stopping the consumption of alcohol can also be extremely effective in treating this group of disorders. With sleepwalkers, particularly children, it is extremely important that the child's room and house be made safe for them if they sleepwalk—they could wander out of their room and fall down the stairs, for example. In general, drug treatment is not recommend unless the person is doing something that will harm themselves or others and they cannot be managed by simpler measures.

> With sleepwalkers, particularly children, it is extremely important that the child's room and house be made safe for them if they sleepwalk

TEETH-GRINDING OR BRUXISM

There are two incarnations of this disorder: While you are sleeping, your upper and lower teeth rapidly grind together, or you clench your jaw. Doctors don't understand why this happens, and in some people it only happens when they are under stress.

WHAT ARE THE SYMPTOMS?

If your bed partner says you sound like a chipmunk when you are sleeping and that you make a noise that is high-pitched and annoying, you wake up with soreness in front of your ears (this is the TMJ, or temporomandibular joint), or your jaw muscles are painful or stiff when you wake up, then you are probably grinding your teeth. This probably happens most commonly when you are under stress (e.g., before an exam or an important interview). Your dentist may also notice that your teeth look like they are being ground down and will tell you during a routine exam that you are grinding your teeth.

CAN ANYTHING STOP TEETH-GRINDING?

This is a problem best assessed and handled by your dentist. One possible treatment is for your dentist to make a mouthguard for you that will help preserve your teeth, as some people may grind their teeth all the way down and lose many teeth.

DSPS AND ASPS

Some people's biological clock is out of sync with what is usual. Those suffering from delayed sleep phase syndrome (DSPS) and advanced sleep phase syndrome (ASPS) sleep and wake at inconvenient times. Individuals with ASPS sleep earlier than their desired clock time, while DSPS sufferers find sleep elusive for hours after their desired clock time. Trying to sleep when their bodies are alert, or to rise when their bodies are sleepiest, can lead to insomnia or excessive daytime sleepiness. Individuals may rely on sleeping pills or alcohol to manipulate their sleep schedules.

HOW DO I KNOW IF I HAVE IT?

DSPS patients may appear to be suffering from insomnia, especially if they insist on trying to sleep at a "normal" bedtime. One distinguishing characteristic is that in other types of insomnia, sleep problems include that of maintaining sleep throughout the night. DSPS sufferers have no problem sleeping—if they observe their own schedules. Another distinction is that most chronic insomniacs experience variability in their nighttime experiences. This is not the case for DSPS patients.

ASPS may be confused with depression. While ASPS appears to be a rare condition, it is more common in seniors. Complaints of difficulty staying awake in evening social situations are one marker of ASPS. Insomnia at the end of the sleep period is another.

> Individuals with ASPS sleep earlier than their desired clock time, while DSPS sufferers find sleep elusive for hours after their desired clock time.

WHAT KIND OF TREATMENT IS THERE?

Treatment of DSPS requires "resetting" the biological clock by using bright light exposure, medication, or chronotherapy. Chronotherapy involves delaying bedtime by three hours progressively each day until the desired bedtime is reached.

Although difficult to accomplish, this approach can work if individuals can alter their schedules daily and protect their sleep from interruptions. Exposure to bright light early in the morning (6 to 9 a.m.) induces a phase advance, leading to an earlier sleep onset that evening. However, individuals must avoid bright light exposure during the evening, as this would tend to delay sleep onset.

Medication is another option. Hypnotics and melatonin may help, but many questions remain about their duration of use and the long-term safety of melatonin. (See Chapter Eight for more on hypnotics and melatonin.)

Treatment for ASPS includes bright light therapy and chronotherapy. The three-hour phase advancement of chronotherapy is implemented every other day. The bright light exposure is usually scheduled for late afternoon or evening.

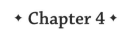

◆ Chapter 4 ◆

Travel, Shift Work,

AND
YOUR PERSONAL
BODY CLOCK

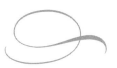

EVEN IF YOU DON'T HAVE ONE of the sleep disorders discussed in the previous chapter, there are still many issues you can have with sleep. In Chapter One, we discussed the existence of the master body clock that regulates when it is time for our bodies to be awake and when it is time for us to be asleep. The body clock likes to keep a regular routine. When we quickly change time zones or sleep when it's daylight and try to stay awake all night, the master body clock will be at odds with our schedule. Sometimes, the internal body clock is broken, and needs to be adjusted to get in sync with what might be considered "regular" hours for sleep and wakefulness. This chapter talks about how we confuse our body clocks and how to deal with body clocks that may be a little off the normal schedule.

TRAVELING BY CAR

THE COMMUTE

Many people who drive to work are tired before they ever get behind the wheel. As the average commute becomes longer and longer, people are driving for long periods of time while being very sleep deprived. Driving drowsy is dangerous. If you space out for one second at sixty miles per hour you will have traveled eighty-eight feet. There are thousands of drowsy driving collisions each year. People should only drive when they've had enough sleep so that they can drive safely. Drinking coffee can help, but it may take fifteen to thirty minutes for the coffee to work and the effect of coffee will wear off rapidly.

If you space out for one second at sixty miles per hour you will have traveled eighty-eight feet.

A LONGER TRIP

Longer trips, whether they are business trips or vacations, require planning. Some people will get up extremely early in the morning to avoid rush hour. Make sure that you have enough sleep before embarking on such a trip. After two hours of driving you should stop every one hundred miles. Get out of the car and at the very least walk around; this will help awaken your brain and will also help prevent blood clots from forming in your legs.

Switch drivers every two to four hours. If you are still sleepy, stop driving, pull into a rest area, and take a fifteen- to thirty-minute nap. You might consider drinking a cup of coffee before the nap so that by the time you wake up, the effects of the nap and the coffee will be working together. Do not drink excessive amounts of coffee the day you are driving, however, because that may disturb the following night's sleep and may cause severe sleepiness on the following day.

JET LAG

Jet lag occurs when you go from one time zone to another fairly quickly and try to sleep or be awake at different times than your body clock expects. Jet lag is much more obvious and disruptive when you cross several time zones and the effects also depend on which direction you are going. It takes a few days for the body clock to adjust completely to the new location. Of course, jet lag does not occur if you fly north or south and stay in the same time zone.

Some symptoms of jet lag can occur if you cross time zones even by car, because it takes several days for the body clock to readjust to the new location. Thus, if you make a rapid cross-country trip from New York to California, you might find yourself waking up in California much earlier than you normally do.

Superimposed on the confusion of when to sleep and when to stay awake is the fact that very often when you change time zones, for example by flying, you will also lose sleep. Thus, there are two things to deal with when you reach your destination: first is that you are often sleep deprived and second is that you may be trying to stay awake at a time when your body clock and brain wants you to sleep, or you are trying to sleep at a time when your body clock expects you to be wide awake.

GENERAL RULES FOR COMBATING JET LAG

Check the time at your destination

First, check the time at your final destination to get a good idea of how many hours you will be shifting. Do not plan any important business for the few hours immediately after arrival at your final destination. If you have really important business to attend to at your destination, try to plan it for a couple of days after you arrive so you will be as mentally sharp as possible.

Reserve a sleep-friendly hotel room

When you make your room reservation, tell them you want a quiet room, away from elevators, ice machines, the laundry, and street noise. Also, this is a good time to tell them you want non-allergenic pillows.

Prepare a sleep kit

Prepare for yourself a little sleep kit containing earplugs or noise cancellation headphones, nasal strips (which can be purchased in a drug store), and an eye mask, which can be found in this kit. Some noise cancellation headphones do not even need to be plugged into an electronic device to cancel noise.

> Do not plan any important business for the few hours immediately after arrival at your final destination.

Check your airline seats

When reserving airline seats, try to get a seat away from the bathrooms or the galleys. These places tend to be very noisy on airplanes. If you can afford it, some airlines now offer seats in business class or higher that can lie flat and become almost enclosed sleeping areas. Decide whether you sleep better in an aisle seat or window seat. Being in the middle is generally not great for sleeping if you are traveling alone.

Set up your sleep environment when you get on the plane

When you get on the airplane, set up your virtual sleep cocoon. You want to be able to block light and noise and be as comfortable as possible. First, let the staff know you do not want to be woken up. Try to get a pillow and/or blanket from the flight attendant. Put on your headphones or earplugs. If you snore, try using nasal strips. Put on the eye mask. You are now in your own personal sleep cocoon.

After you arrive, check your room

When you check into the hotel, ensure that you do indeed have a "quiet" room. Then check to see whether the pillows are suitable for you and whether the mattress is comfortable. Next, check the noise from the air-handling system, noise from outside the hotel, and if you are near an airport, listen carefully to make sure that you're not near a flight path. Being away from elevators is also a good general rule because some elevators will make a sound whenever the elevator arrives at the floor, and again when the doors open and close. Also make sure that the room has light-blocking curtains, and that you can control the temperature.

A quick trip idea

If you are doing a quick trip and plan to return immediately after your business, you might try not shifting your body clock at all and making your travel arrangements in such a way that you can return to your home destination quickly. For example, imagine you are flying to London from New York City. You check the time difference and you notice that it is five hours. Your flight leaves at 8 p.m., and you land at 6 a.m. London-time. Your body clock when you land will think that it is 1 a.m. You certainly wouldn't want to schedule a meeting at 9 a.m. London-time, because your brain will still think that it is the middle of the night, and you will probably be dead tired. In that type of situation, plan your important business meeting for the early afternoon, or even mid-afternoon. By then, your body clock will expect you to be awake, and you will be naturally more alert. But when do you sleep? In that situation, some experienced business travelers would stay awake until about their normal sleep time, and sleep only a couple of hours on the flight. When they arrived in London, they would go to their hotel and immediately take a nap to catch up on lost sleep. On the ride from the airport to the hotel, they would wear sunglasses so as not to confuse their body clock, which is already beginning to wonder where they are.

TIPS FOR FLYING

→ **A short trip flying east crossing three time zones (e.g., Los Angeles to New York City)**

- Do not plan important meetings for the first couple of mornings
- Avoid red-eye flights

→ **A long trip flying east crossing five or more time zones (e.g., New York City to Paris)**

Suppose your flight leaves at 9:30 p.m. New York-time, which is 3:30 a.m. Paris-time. After the seven-hour flight, your body will think it is 4:30 a.m., but it is actually 10:30 a.m. in Paris. Thus, your brain will be confused for two reasons—it has lost sleep and it is confused about what time it is. These are some of the rules that you can follow to help combat the problems of jet lag:

- First, if you're planning to take any sleeping pills or products such as melatonin, do not take them unless you're 100 percent certain that the airplane is actually going to be taking off. The last thing you want to do is take something that will make you fall asleep, but then not travel on the airplane.

- When you get on the airplane, tell the flight attendant that you do not want to be woken up during the night. You do not want to be told about extra meals or movies and only want to be woken up before landing. Avoid any alcohol. Drink plenty of fluids before you try to sleep.

- Do everything you can to try to help induce sleep. Use earplugs or noise cancellation headphones and an eye mask and cover yourself with a blanket. If you snore, try nasal strips. You may sleep more deeply and your neighbors will appreciate the quiet.

- Once you are airborne, the strategy is to fall asleep at the same time as people are falling asleep at your destination. On this eastward trip, when you get onto the airplane, most people at your destination are already asleep, so you should try to fall asleep as soon as you can. Some people will use sleep aids such as sleeping pills or melatonin. If you are prescribed a sleep aid, make sure it is a short acting one. You do not want to be in a daze when you land. Absolutely do not use alcohol to fall asleep because alcohol actually disrupts your sleep.

- What you are trying to accomplish is to switch over to the sleep-wake pattern of your destination, so it is best that you not eat a meal during the middle of the flight. Anyway, it will be much more exciting to have your first meal in a French café, munching on a fresh baguette, or warm croissants, with a delicious café au lait. This will also help you wake up.

- On the way to the hotel, do not wear sunglasses. Exposure to sunlight will help your body clock readjust more quickly.

→ **A long trip flying west crossing five or six time zones (e.g., Berlin to Philadelphia)**

If you are flying from Berlin to Philadelphia (a seven-hour flight), the flight usually leaves in the morning and you will travel most of the day in sunlight.

- It is best to take a short nap, perhaps an hour or so.

- Try to stay awake until roughly the normal bedtime of your new destination.

- Watch the movies.

- Eat what they give you.

- Avoid alcohol.

- You will be extremely tired when you arrive and you will have an excellent sleep that night. You may, however, wake up early. These early awakenings may continue for several days.

→ **A long trip flying west crossing seven or more time zones (e.g., San Francisco to Tokyo)**

These flights frequently leave around noontime, but it is already bedtime in your destination when you take off.

- Try to sleep right away.

- Try to spend five to seven hours sleeping.

- After sleeping, watch the movies, eat the food, and try to stay awake.

- By the time you land, clear customs, and take the train from the airport to the city, it will be evening and you will be very tired, but try to stay awake as long as you can. When you go to sleep you will sleep deeply, but it is very likely you will awaken early in the morning. Your body clock has not yet adjusted. A wonderful thing to do that first morning in Tokyo is to go to the fish market. It is open very early in the morning and you'll enjoy the hustle and bustle and some delicious sushi.

→ **Flying to the other side of the world**

Since there are only twenty-four time zones, you cannot be more than twelve time zones away from your final destination. If you are traveling such a great number of time zones, it doesn't really matter whether you're traveling east or west, although psychologically people may react differently.

- When traveling through so many time zones, try to use the rules mentioned above for more than five time zones, but bear in mind that it will take much longer to adjust at your final destination, and it will be much tougher to readjust back when you return home.

A QUICK SUMMARY OF ADJUSTING TO JET LAG

There are two components to combating jet lag. First, try to get as much sleep as you can to combat the sleep deprivation that accompanies jet lag. Second, help your body clock adjust to your new destination.

To help you adjust:

- Do not expect to adjust quickly.

- Make sure that you switch to the sleep-wake schedule of your destination as quickly as possible after arrival.

- Try to avoid very long naps during the daytime as you are adjusting.

- Make sure you do not use excessive amounts of caffeine to try to maintain alertness, since that will make it much more difficult to sleep at night.

- Do not expect to be mentally sharp for the first few days after a long flight over many time zones.

- Expect up to one day of not being 100 percent for every time zone that you have crossed. Some people who adjust much more quickly will be at 100 percent in two to three days, no matter how many time zones they have crossed.

Bon Voyage!

SHIFT WORK

Do you work at times other than the usual "nine-to-five" business day? If so, you are among the millions of shift workers in America's workplace. You may work when most people are asleep and attempt to sleep when the rest of the world is awake. Shift workers perform critical functions in hospitals, on police forces, as emergency personnel, and in the transportation and manufacturing industries. In addition, they are meeting the demand for "round-the-clock" service in an age of global interaction. More than 15 million Americans are shift workers.

Unfortunately, when it comes to sleep, most shift workers don't get enough. When shifts fall during the night (11 p.m. to 7 a.m.) the worker fights his or her natural wake-sleep pattern. It may be hard to stay alert at night and just as hard to fall asleep and stay asleep during the day. Night workers typically get less sleep than daytime workers do, and the sleep is less restful. As we have already learned, sleep is more than just "beauty rest" for the body; it helps restore and rejuvenate the brain and organ systems so that they function properly.

Some of the most serious and persistent problems shift workers face are frequent sleep disturbance and associated excessive sleepiness. Fatigue in the workplace can lead to poor concentration, absenteeism, accidents, errors, injuries, and fatalities. The issue becomes more alarming when you consider that shift workers are often employed in the most dangerous of jobs, such as firefighting, emergency medical services, law enforcement, and security. Although addressing these issues may require some investment up front for training and other measures, the bottom line is that improved sleep in workers may lead to improved productivity. In fact, to ignore the needs of the shift worker is reckless and irresponsible when you consider that billions of dollars in yearly costs, thousands of deaths, and some of the most notorious of modern catastrophes such as the nuclear meltdown at Three Mile Island and the ecological disaster caused by the oil spill of the Exxon Valdez oil tanker have been partially attributed to human fatigue.

Modern catastrophes such as the nuclear meltdown at Three Mile Island and the ecological disaster caused by the oil spill of the Exxon Valdez oil tanker have been partially attributed to human fatigue.

SUCCESSFUL SHUT-EYE!

There are several steps a shift worker can take to successfully fall asleep and stay asleep (see the tips below). The key is to make sleep a priority! Set the stage for sleep even though it might be broad daylight outside. Prepare your body and mind for sleep. If you are on the night shift, wear wrap-around dark glasses on your way home from work to keep morning sunlight from activating your internal "daytime" clock. Follow bedtime rituals and try to keep the same sleep schedule—even on weekends or days off. Go to sleep as soon as possible after work. At home, ask family and friends to help create a quiet and peaceful setting during your sleep time. Have family members wear headphones to listen to music or watch TV. Ban vacuuming, dish washing, and noisy games during your sleep time. Schedule household deliveries and repairs for after your sleep time.

TIPS FOR THE SHIFT WORKER

→ **Bedtime Rituals**

- Take a warm bath.

- Lower the room temperature (a cool environment improves sleep).

- Don't stimulate your brain in bed by reading a thriller or doing any other stressful activities.

→ **Light**

- Darken the bedroom and bathroom.

- Install light blocking and sound absorbing curtains and shades.

- Wear eye shades or an eye mask such as the one included in this kit.

→ **Sound**

- Wear ear plugs.

- Use a white noise machine or a fan to block out noises.

- Install carpeting and drapes to absorb sound.

- Mute the phones.

→ **Food**

- Avoid caffeine at least five hours before bedtime.

- Don't stop for a drink after work—alcohol disturbs sleep.

- Eat a light snack—don't go to bed too full or too hungry.

→ **Exercise**

- Exercise after you wake up from your sleep—exercise is alerting and raises your body temperature.

THE RIDE HOME

Driving home after work can be risky for a shift worker, particularly since you have been awake all night and your body needs to sleep. For the evening worker coming home around midnight, the risk of meeting drunk drivers is higher. People think that opening the car windows or listening to the radio will keep them awake, however, studies show that these methods do not work. In fact, these actions should signal to you that you are fatigued and need to pull over and rest. If you are sleepy when your shift is over, try to take a fifteen- to twenty-minute nap before driving home. Sleep can quickly overcome you when you don't want it to!

TIPS FOR THE RIDE HOME

→ **Arriving Home Safely From Your Shift**

- Carpool, if possible. Have the most alert person do the driving.

- If you are sleepy, stop to nap, but do so in your locked car in a well-lit area.

- Take public transportation, if possible.

- Drive defensively.

- Don't stop off for a "night cap."

> If you are sleepy when your shift is over, try to take a fifteen- to twenty-minute nap before driving home.

UNDERSTANDING YOUR BODY CLOCK

Shift work has become an indispensable part of modern life and many people can successfully adapt and be productive. The body clock has a powerful effect on when we sleep and when we are awake and alert, and many of the things we do such as travel, work, and play are at odds with the clock. Understanding how to adjust to the realities of modern life will help us get the most out of our twenty-four-hour day.

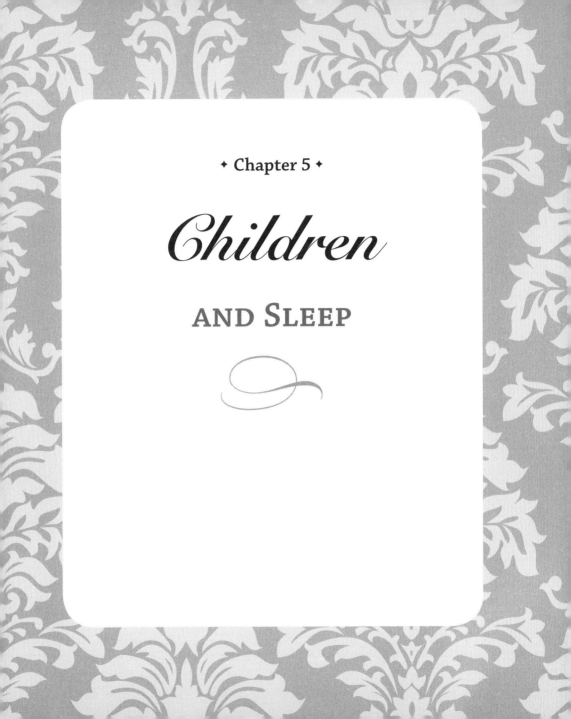

◆ Chapter 5 ◆

Children

AND SLEEP

IF YOU HAVE CHILDREN, YOU MAY be familiar with their sleepless nights. Twenty-five percent of kids experience a sleep problem at some point during childhood, and when your kids aren't sleeping, YOU aren't sleeping. Unfortunately, sleep problems in children can be chronic and bad habits can be difficult for parents to break once established. The good news, however, is that sleep problems in children are highly treatable. Make sleeping through the night a priority for your child, yourself, and your family.

SLEEP AND DEVELOPMENT IN CHILDREN

In Chapter One, we learned that sleep is a vital need for everyone, but it is especially important for children as it directly impacts mental and physical development. Sleep is essential for a child's health, growth, and proper development. Sleep promotes alertness, learning, performance, and even good behavior. It is the primary activity of the brain during early development. As we learned in Chapter Two, circadian rhythms, or the sleep-wake cycle, are regulated by light and dark and these rhythms take time to develop, resulting in the irregular sleep schedules of newborns. By the age of two, most children have spent more time asleep than awake.

Because sleep is so essential to a child's development, it is important for parents to begin helping their children develop high-quality sleep habits as early as possible. Here is the chart we saw earlier to remind you how many hours of sleep babies and children need:

HOW MUCH SLEEP DO YOU REALLY NEED?	
AGE	**SLEEP NEEDS**
Newborns (1–2 months)	10.5–18 hours
Infants (3–11 months)	9–12 hours at night and 30-minute–2-hour naps, 1–4 times per day
Toddlers (1–3 years)	12–14 hours
Preschoolers (3–5 years)	11–13 hours
Children (5–12 years)	10–11 hours
Teens (13–17 years)	8.5–9.25 hours
Adults	7–9 hours
Older Adults	7–9 hours

Besides getting enough sleep, children need to learn healthy sleep habits at an early age. Once established, these habits will serve them well into adolescence and adulthood.

FOUR WAYS TO DEVELOP HEALTHY SLEEP HABITS IN CHILDREN

- Make bedtime the same time every night.

- Make your child's bedtime routine a positive and relaxing experience. Save your child's favorite relaxing activities, such as reading a story, until last and have them occur in the child's bedroom.

- Make your child's bedroom sleep-friendly—cool, dark, quiet, and comfortable. Televisions, computers, cell phones, hand-held computer games, and all other electronics should be relegated to another room of the house. Studies clearly show that electronics in the bedroom make it harder for children to get the sleep they need and contribute to sleep problems.

- Encourage children to fall asleep on their own. Children can learn to self-soothe and not rely on a parent to help them fall asleep. The child who falls asleep on his or her own will be better able to return to sleep following normal nighttime awakenings and thus, sleep throughout the night.

FOR NEW MOTHERS

Babies should be put to sleep on their backs. According to the "Back to Sleep" program, this lowers the risk of death from Sudden Infant Death Syndrome (SIDS). The American Academy of Pediatrics also recommends that parents should avoid placing young children to sleep on a water bed, sofa, pillow, soft mattress, or other soft surfaces.

During the first few months, sleep when your baby sleeps. A well-rested mom can make all the difference in dealing successfully with the stressors of a new baby in the house.

For young children, naptime and nighttime sleep are both necessary and independent of each other. Children who consistently nap are usually less cranky and sleep better at night. It is important not to stop naps at too young an age. Don't be surprised, though, if there comes a time that your child still clearly needs his or her nap but the napping makes it more difficult for him or her to fall asleep at bedtime. This will occur when your child is transitioning away from naps, often between the ages of three and five.

A well-rested mom can make all the difference in dealing successfully with the stressors of a new baby in the house.

TIPS FOR INFANTS

→ **Newborn to twelve months**

- Establish a regular sleep schedule for your baby.

- Put your baby to sleep on his or her back.

- Create a consistent and enjoyable bedtime routine.

- Avoid feeding your baby to sleep. Try to give your baby a bottle or nurse earlier in the evening. Do not put your baby to sleep with a bottle.

- Put your baby to bed drowsy but awake, and encourage him or her to fall asleep independently.

→ **12 months to 3 years**

- Maintain a daily sleep schedule with regular naptimes and bedtime.
- Establish a consistent bedtime routine.
- Make the bedroom environment the same every night and throughout the night.
- Put your toddler to bed drowsy but awake.
- Set limits that are consistent and enforced.
- Encourage use of a security object, such as a blanket or stuffed animal.

For fun activities to help your children learn about healthy sleep habits, visit the National Sleep Foundation Web site for kids, www.sleepforkids.com. There you will find activities, games, and puzzles that can help teach your children about the importance of sleep and make bedtime a great time for your kids!

SLEEP PROBLEMS IN CHILDREN

Some sleep problems occur more frequently in children than adults. This can include problems such as nightmares, sleepwalking, and bedwetting. Additionally, kids are not immune to some of the same serious sleep disorders that afflict adults. One of the main symptoms of sleep problems in children is that they begin to have problems in school; often they become inattentive or actually nod off. Falling asleep in school is never caused by not eating breakfast! It is always caused by sleep deprivation, poor quality sleep, or a sleep disorder. Sometimes the sleepiness in school may be caused by medications used to treat another medical condition.

Let's take a moment to look at some of these problems and discuss tips to get your kids back on track to a good night's sleep.

> One of the main symptoms of sleep problems in children is that they begin to have problems in school; often they become inattentive or actually nod off.

NIGHTMARES

Nightmares often occur at times of transition, stress, or change in a child's routine. They usually take place later in the night and are remembered the next day. Fortunately, nightmares tend to go away naturally. Encouraging your child to talk about the nightmare, discussing comforting images before lights out, and avoiding television immediately before bedtime are strategies that assist in alleviating nightmares.

BEDWETTING

Bedwetting is very common during the toilet-training years. If a child continues to wet the bed more than twice a month after age six or seven, you should consider consulting a pediatrician. Prior to that age, many children continue to have problems staying dry through the night. Bedwetting in older children may simply be a result of immaturity. However, it may be an indication of an underlying medical condition.

SLEEP TERROR

Sleep terror and/or sleepwalking occur most frequently from four to eight years of age. These sleep disruptions occur during the early part of the night. During an episode of sleep terror, your child may scream and appear to be frightened or aggressive but he or she is actually asleep. Your child is both asleep and awake at the same time during these episodes and often has no memory of the event the next day. Waking or comforting your child is usually not helpful as it prolongs the event. It is best just to quietly lead the child back to bed. There is no advantage to discussing or describing these episodes the next day, since this may lead to greater stress in the child and result in a fear of going to sleep. Often these episodes are more common in sleep-deprived children, and when they sleep enough, the episodes may go away. Be sure both your child's room and your house are safe.

IS IT ADHD, SLEEP DEPRIVATION, OR BOTH?

Attention-Deficit/Hyperactivity Disorder (ADHD) is a distinct disorder; however, research has shown that some children may be misdiagnosed with ADHD when the real problem is chronic sleep deprivation due to a sleep disorder or poor sleeping habits. A number of pediatric sleep specialists are concerned that children who are being misdiagnosed with ADHD are being put on medication without first assessing for sleep problems. In addition, studies show that individuals who do in fact have ADHD also often suffer from sleep disorders such as sleep apnea, insomnia, or restless legs syndrome. In many cases, children who have both ADHD and a sleep disorder have shown marked improvement in their symptoms after the sleep problem is treated. If you have concerns about your child's sleep and he or she has been diagnosed with ADHD, speak to your pediatrician or a pediatric sleep specialist to determine if lack of sleep could be part of the problem.

SLEEP DISORDERS IN CHILDREN

SLEEP APNEA

Yes, children can have sleep apnea, and it is more common than was previously thought. Children with sleep apnea may snore and be observed to gasp or stop breathing, or they may have restless sleep. Sometimes they will sleep with their head in an unusual position in an attempt to keep their breathing passage open. In 2002 the American Academy of Pediatrics recommended that all children who snore be evaluated to rule out sleep apnea. Most of the time enlarged tonsils and adenoids, small jaws, and/or obesity account for sleep apnea in children. For enlarged tonsils and adenoids, children should be evaluated by an ear, nose, and throat specialist. If a child has a very small jaw, they should be assessed by an orthodontist before they have stopped growing (preferably before the ages of twelve to fourteen). Childhood obesity, which is becoming a public health problem, could also be the cause of sleep apnea in children. Seek help early if a child has sleep apnea because of obesity.

RESTLESS LEGS SYNDROME

Restless Legs Syndrome (RLS) affects approximately 2 percent of children. As we learned in Chapter Three it is a neurological disorder that causes unpleasant sensations in the legs, usually while at rest and at night. Children with RLS will feel compelled to move or kick their legs to relieve the uncomfortable sensations. This can be very frustrating for the parent and child when trying to settle down and is obviously disruptive to falling asleep.

NARCOLEPSY

Narcolepsy (see Chapter Three for details) is often first noticed following puberty, but may occur as early as ten years of age, or sometimes even earlier. Children with narcolepsy experience excessive daytime sleepiness and uncontrollable "sleep attacks," even when they get enough sleep. Often the first clue is a drop in school performance. They also may have very frightening dream imagery as they fall asleep.

TREATMENT

If your child is experiencing sleep problems or you suspect a sleep disorder such as sleep apnea, RLS, or narcolepsy, you should consult your pediatrician or a sleep specialist for assessment, diagnosis, and treatment.

A WORD ON TEENAGERS

In the case of teenagers, the story is a bit different. A 2007 National Sleep Foundation survey on adolescents' sleep habits and patterns revealed that as many as 60 percent of middle and high school students are sleepy during the day. This is again almost always a matter of inadequate and/or irregular sleep patterns and not so much the cause of sleep disorders. Sleep deprivation is often due to a number of lifestyle and environmental issues. A teenager's biological tendency and lifestyle often result in going to bed too late. They are often up until 1:00 a.m. studying or playing on the computer. Then they are forced to wake up for school, often at an hour that is considered too early by many sleep experts, who point out that adolescents' internal clocks lead to a delay in sleep and wake times. How can they possibly be getting enough sleep? In more severe situations, adolescents develop delayed sleep phase syndrome (see Chapter Four), where their sleep-wake schedule prevents them from going to school or doing other activities on a regular daily schedule. This leads to enormous stress in the family as adults come in conflict with the adolescent about his or her schedule, often resulting in school difficulties as the student becomes chronically late or falls asleep during the early part of the school day. Such teenagers are also at risk to fall asleep while driving. Educating the educators about this might lead the school to accommodate the teenager's schedule and this can lead to a very favorable conclusion. You might have to get a doctor to contact the school to explain the problem.

A 2007 National Sleep Foundation survey on adolescents' sleep habits and patterns revealed that as many as 60 percent of middle and high school students are sleepy during the day.

AWARENESS OF SLEEP ISSUES IN CHILDREN

Sleep deprivation is very common in younger people and should be addressed. If there is a disorder present, it can often be diagnosed at a young age and will hopefully be treated sooner rather than later. While some disorders are more common in children, others can show up at any time. It is important to be aware of your child's sleep patterns and try to acclimate them to a healthy sleep schedule early in life so they will always be able to feel good and be healthy.

◆ Chapter 6 ◆

Sleep

AND AGING

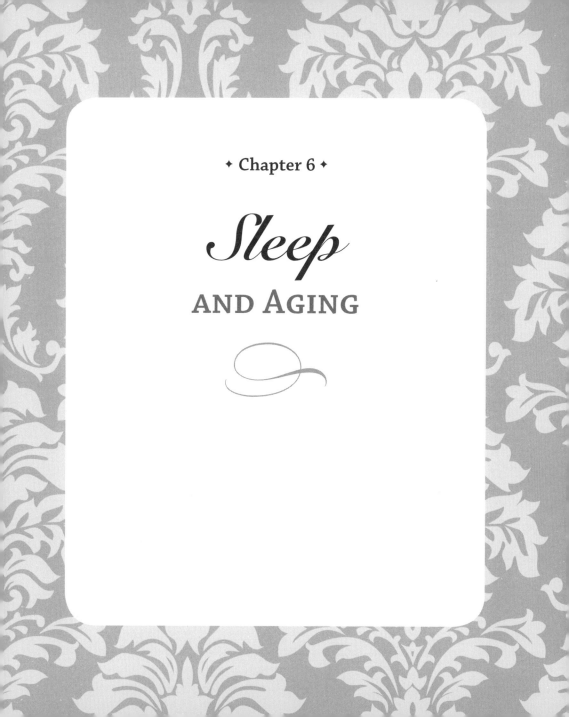

THE CHANGES THAT AGING BRINGS tend to come upon us unnoticed at first, like the passing of the seasons. Slowly, over time, we become aware that our eyesight is less keen or our hearing less acute. In a similar fashion, our experience of sleep changes too—and often for the worse. Along with the physical changes that occur as we get older, changes to our sleep patterns are also a part of the normal aging process. As we age, we tend to have a harder time falling asleep and more trouble staying asleep than when we were younger. This may sound familiar to you from Chapter Three, where we covered insomnia. It is a common misconception that sleep needs decline with age. In fact, research demonstrates that our sleep needs remain constant throughout adulthood. Again, seven to nine hours of sleep seems to be optimal for most adults—aging or not.

CHANGES IN SLEEP ARCHITECTURE

So, what's keeping seniors awake? Changes in the patterns of our sleep—what specialists call "sleep architecture"—occur as we age and this may contribute to sleep problems. As you may recall from Chapter One, sleep occurs in multiple stages, including dreamless periods of light and deep sleep, and occasional periods of active dreaming (REM sleep). The sleep cycle is repeated several times during the night and although total sleep time tends to remain constant, older people spend more time in the lighter stages of sleep (stages 1 and 2) rather than in deep sleep (stages 3 and 4).

Many older adults, though certainly not all, also report being less satisfied with sleep and feel more tired during the day. Studies on the sleep habits of older Americans show an increase in the time it takes to fall asleep, an overall decline in REM sleep, and an increase in sleep fragmentation (waking up during the night) with age. The prevalence of sleep disorders also tends to increase with age. However, research suggests that much of the sleep disturbance among older adults can be attributed to physical and psychiatric illnesses and the medications used to treat them.

HOW SLEEP CHANGES AS WE AGE

+ The time spent in various stages of sleep shifts from more time in deep sleep to more time in lighter sleep.
+ Nighttime sleep is more likely to be disturbed.
+ Medical conditions are more prevalent in older people and can adversely affect sleep quality and duration.
+ Older people tend to nap more than younger adults.

The National Sleep Foundation 2003 Sleep in America Poll profiled the sleep patterns and sleep complaints of 1,506 older Americans. About two-thirds of older adults (67 percent) reported experiencing one or more of the following symptoms of a sleep problem at least a few nights a week:

+ difficulty falling asleep
+ waking a lot during the night
+ waking up early and not being able to get back to sleep
+ waking up feeling unrefreshed
+ snoring
+ pauses in breathing
+ unpleasant feelings in their legs

In spite of the abundance of these sleep complaints, only a small fraction (one out of eight) said that they had been diagnosed with a sleep disorder and even fewer were treated.

CHANGES IN CIRCADIAN RHYTHM

In addition to changes in sleep architecture that occur as we age, other factors affecting our sleep are the circadian rhythms that coordinate the timing of our bodily functions, including sleep. Recall our discussion of the master clock in Chapter One and the broken body clock in Chapter Four. For example, older people tend to become sleepier in the early evening and wake earlier in the morning compared to younger adults. The sleep rhythm is shifted forward so that seven or eight hours of sleep are still obtained, but the individuals will wake up extremely early because they have gone to sleep so early. The reason for these changes in sleep and circadian rhythms as we age is not clearly understood.

→ **"I was giving a lecture to a group of older people when a woman told me that she woke up at 4 a.m. and was very upset and wanted sleeping pills. I asked two questions. First, when did she go to sleep? And second, how did she feel during the daytime? The answer to the first was '8 p.m.' and the answer to the second was 'Great.' She was eating the 'early bird' supper at a restaurant every day at 4 p.m. The person's body clock was running about two to three hours early."**

→   **—Dr. Meir Kryger**

WHAT CAUSES SLEEP DIFFICULTIES IN OLDER PEOPLE?

Older adults generally secrete lesser amounts of hormones that help regulate the sleep-wake cycle. Both melatonin and growth hormone production decrease with age. There are also changes in the body temperature cycle that occur with age. These factors may cause, or be a consequence of, sleep problems. In addition, a decrease in exposure to natural light and a change in diet may exacerbate sleep difficulties. Some researchers theorize that daytime inactivity and decreased mental stimulation may also lead to the "aging" of sleep.

Falling asleep isn't the only difficulty older individuals may face at night. Sleep also becomes more shallow, fragmented, and variable in duration with age. Older adults wake more frequently than younger adults. The aging bladder or an enlarged prostate in men may also contribute to nighttime awakenings. It is important to remember, however, that persistent trouble falling asleep at night or frequent drowsiness by day is not normal or inevitable with age.

> Persistent trouble falling asleep at night or frequent drowsiness by day is not normal or inevitable with age.

As we age, there is an increased incidence of medical problems, which are often chronic. In general, people with poor health or chronic medical conditions have more sleep problems. For example, hypertension is associated with both snoring and obstructive sleep apnea (OSA) and heart failure, which affect approximately 5 million Americans. In addition, menopause and its accompanying hot flashes, night sweats, changes in breathing, and decreasing hormone levels can lead to many restless nights for women.

Medical conditions such as diabetes mellitus, renal failure, respiratory diseases such as asthma, and immune disorders are all associated with sleep problems. Diseases such as depression, Parkinson's disease, and multiple sclerosis also commonly cause problems sleeping.

SLEEP APNEA IN THE OLDER PERSON

As mentioned in Chapter Three, sleep apnea occurs in approximately 4 to 5 percent of the population. However, in males over sixty-five, the figure rises to 28 percent and for women, the number climbs to 24 percent. Again, sleep apnea is a serious sleep disorder that is treatable. Refer to Chapter Three for a discussion of treatment options.

INSOMNIA IN THE OLDER PERSON

In most people, insomnia is a chronic problem and so it is not surprising that insomnia is very common in older people. In general, the more medical conditions present, the more likely insomnia will be a problem. Sometimes medications that older people are taking may cause insomnia. There are two facts to remember about insomnia in older people: first, older people are very sensitive to medications and thus a dose of a sleeping pill that might be appropriate for a younger adult may have significant side effects, for example confusion at night if they awaken or a "hangover" in the morning. Second, older people with insomnia should pay particular attention to napping. Naps should be kept to no more than 30 to 45 minutes, or they should be avoided entirely.

NARCOLEPSY IN THE OLDER PERSON

Although narcolepsy usually begins in the teenage years, it is often not diagnosed until ten to fifteen years after the symptoms of sleepiness begin. There are patients whose narcolepsy was first diagnosed when they were in their sixties. These unfortunate people were often labeled as lazy and spent almost an entire lifetime in the fog of sleepiness. Their lives might have been much different had they been diagnosed and treated when they were teenagers. Because narcolepsy is a chronic condition, people treated for this condition in their younger years will still require treatment. Sometimes medications used to treat sleepiness may be a problem if the patient develops heart disease.

SPOTLIGHT ON ALZHEIMER'S DISEASE

One of the many side effects of Alzheimer's disease, as well as other forms of dementia, is that the disease has negative effects on the sleep-wake cycle. The greater the degree of dementia, the sleepier the patient is. With more severe forms of dementia, patients are often sleepier during the day, and their sleep at night tends to be fragmented and disrupted. Over a twenty-four-hour period, for example, patients are rarely awake and rarely asleep for a full hour at a time. They are constantly waking up at night and falling asleep during the day. This pattern is fairly common in Alzheimer's patients.

Fortunately, there are some things you as a caretaker can do at home to help improve the patient's behavior:

✦ Keep the patient on as regular a schedule as possible. Get him or her out of bed at the same time each morning, and put him or her to bed at the same time each night. Try to discourage him or her from taking multiple naps during the day—one nap in the afternoon is all right, as long as it lasts no more than an hour. During the day, keep the patient as active as possible.

✦ It is also important to get the patient to eat his or her meals at a regular time each day. In fact, the more routine there is in the schedule, the better the patient is able to cope with the effects of Alzheimer's.

✦ It is important to expose the patient to as much bright light as possible. In a nursing home, most patients are exposed to bright light for only ten minutes a day. Even if still living at home, patients are often exposed to sunlight about thirty minutes a day. Even this is not enough. It is better if the patient is exposed to bright light for several hours a day. Take him or her outside whenever possible, especially in the morning. Morning light offers the best exposure, because in a patient with dementia, his or her circadian (biological) rhythm is out of sync with the rhythm of the environment. Bright light improves his or her functioning and makes him or her more alert.

It is also important that the environment be dark at night. If the patient tends to wander at night and you are worried about him or her falling or bumping into furniture, you can keep a nightlight on. But understand that bright light interferes with circadian rhythms. Otherwise, keep the patient's bedroom as dark as possible. You should also keep the environment as quiet as possible during the night.

✦ Avoid feeding the patient caffeine products such as coffee, tea, chocolate, or soda, because they interfere with the circadian rhythm.

✦ Exercise is very important. Have the patient do whatever he or she is capable of doing: for example, take the patient on a short walk every day on a regular basis, and engage him or her in throwing a beach ball. Even if he or she has to use a wheelchair, encourage him or her to do arm exercises.

In addition, one of the characteristics of dementia is sleep disordered breathing. More than 80 percent of dementia patients have sleep apnea. If they can be treated successfully for sleep apnea, their sleep at night and their alertness during the day might be able to be improved. Speak to the patient's physician about this possibility.

Improving sleep at night and functioning during the day helps to postpone institutionalization, which is usually better for the patient and the family.

HELPING SENIORS SLEEP WELL

Although there is a popular myth that all older people will have terrible sleep as they age, this is not true for many. An older healthy person can expect to have normal sleep and expect to be alert in the daytime. Older people who do have sleep problems or who have sleepiness that interferes with their ability to enjoy life should seek help from their doctors. They can usually be helped.

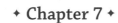

✦ Chapter 7 ✦

Sleeping Pills, Medications,
AND HERBAL REMEDIES

WHEN PEOPLE HAVE TROUBLE SLEEPING, they may turn to prescription drugs, over-the-counter pills, dietary supplements, or herbal remedies in the quest for a good night's sleep. But, with so many options, it can be difficult to know which treatment, if any, is best for you. Sleep aids vary in a number of ways—they act on distinct parts of the brain and differ in their side effects, the length of time they are active in your body, and even in the amount of research required before they can be sold and whether they require a prescription. That's why it is important to know what each type of sleep aid has to offer, and what risks you should watch out for, so you can find the safest treatment that works for you.

USING MEDICATIONS

Not treating a sleep problem can have a negative impact on your safety and overall quality of life, and sometimes medications can be a helpful part of that treatment. In general, sleep medications may be useful when:

+ Insomnia is temporary or short-term.
+ Insomnia is chronic, as outlined in recent NIH recommendations.
+ Insomnia is present with a known health condition (such as pain from arthritis) or an event such as anxiety about giving a speech the next day or traveling across time zones.
+ The explanation of your sleep problem has been identified by your healthcare professional, and he or she decides that it is best treated with medication or a combination of behavioral changes and medication.

Treatment with medications should:

+ Begin with the lowest possible effective dose.
+ Use a medication actually approved by the FDA for initiating sleep (some doctors prescribe psychiatric medications that are not approved for this use).
+ Be short-term (two weeks), if used nightly, although recently the FDA has approved some sleep medications for use up to six months.
+ Be intermittent (three to four nights a week), if used long-term.
+ Be used only in combination with good sleep practices and/or behavioral approaches.
+ Include a plan that involves reassessing the patient to see if the treatment is effective without side effects and a discussion of when the medications might be stopped.

It is important to know what each type of sleep aid has to offer, and what risks you should watch out for, so you can find the safest treatment that works for you.

PRESCRIPTION SLEEPING PILLS

Prescription sleep medications are called hypnotics. These drugs have been well-researched and are FDA-approved to treat insomnia. Studies have shown that hypnotics are reliable for:

+ Shortening the time it takes to fall asleep.
+ Increasing total sleep time.
+ Decreasing the number of nighttime awakenings.
+ Improving sleep quality.

You should never use a medication prescribed for another person.

Hypnotics are usually prescribed for short-term management of sleep problems. They are often just one part of an overall treatment plan that your healthcare provider can tailor to your particular medical history and lifestyle. Hypnotics have unwanted effects in some people, which are described below. You should never use a medication prescribed for another person. You might be surprised to learn that many doctors prescribe medications "off-label." That prescription for a "sleeping pill" that your friend is taking might turn out to be a powerful drug used to treat schizophrenia (which your friend may not even have). Doctors are relying on the side effects of these powerful drugs to help induce sleep. The media has covered stories of celebrities dying of overdose or drug interaction after using medications sometimes not prescribed for them.

How do hypnotics work? Hypnotics act on specific parts of the brain to promote sleep. There are two main types of hypnotics—melatonin receptor agonists and benzodiazepine receptor agonists (BzRAs). There are two types of BzRAs—benzodiazepines and nonbenzodiazepines—and these names simply reflect a difference in their chemical structures (they both promote sleep by acting on benzodiazepine receptors). The chart on the following page shows the only products as of early 2009 approved by the FDA to treat insomnia.

Generic Name	Brand Name	Duration of Action
Ramelteon	Rozerem®	Short
Estazolam	Prosom®	Long
Eszopiclone	Lunesta®	Medium
Flurazepam	Dalmane®	Very long
Quazepam	Doral®	Very long
Temazepam	Restoril®	Long
Triazolam	Halcion®	Short
Zaleplon	Sonata®	Very short
Zolpidem	Ambien®	Short
Zolpidem CR	Ambien CR®	Medium

Melatonin Receptor Agonists

Ramelteon (Rozerem®) acts on melatonin receptors in the brain and is prescribed
to help patients fall asleep more quickly. These receptors act on the body clock
(remember the suprachiasmatic nucleus?) and turn off a signal that arouses the
brain, and thus may help induce sleep. Ramelteon has been approved by the FDA
for long-term use and studies have shown that it does not cause dependence,
abuse, withdrawal, or rebound insomnia. Rebound insomnia happens in some
people when they stop taking a sleeping medication: the insomnia is temporarily

Type of Action	FDA Approved for Short-term Use	FDA Approved for Long-term Use
Melatonin receptor agonist	Yes	Yes
BzRA (benzodiazepine)	Yes	No
BzRA (nonbenzodiazepine)	Yes	Yes
BzRA (benzodiazepine)	Yes	No
BzRA (benzodiazepine)	Yes	No
BzRA (benzodiazepine)	Yes	No
BzRA (benzodiazepine)	Yes	No
BzRA (nonbenzodiazepine)	Yes	No
BzRA (nonbenzodiazepine)	Yes	No
BzRA (nonbenzodiazepine)	Yes	Yes

worse than before they started treatment. This is good news, but it is still unclear whether ramelteon is as effective as BzRAs in treating insomnia for many patients. It is only prescribed to help with sleep onset (as opposed to nighttime awakenings). Ramelteon is generally well-tolerated, but among people who experience side effects, the most common ones are next-day drowsiness, dizziness, and fatigue. Also, studies show that patients won't suffer from memory lapses of events that occur while they are using this medicine.

Benzodiazepine Receptor Agonists (BzRAs)

BzRAs promote sleep by increasing the normal effects of a brain chemical called gamma-amniobutyric acid (GABA). Originally the benzodiazepine receptor agonists were all benzodiazepines, which had other effects on the nervous system, not just on sleep; more recently the medications introduced, which are nonbenzodiazepines, have fewer of these effects on the nervous system. There are a number of BzRAs that doctors can prescribe, and the main difference among them is the length of time they stay active in the body. This allows doctors to select the right medication to match the patient's sleep problem and lifestyle. The pills with a longer duration are more likely to work for the entire night, but they may also make you feel groggy the next morning and can be risky if you need to be "on-call" if you are woken up during the night—for example, if you are caring for a small child or may have to make important decisions upon awakening.

How safe are BzRAs? Research has shown that BzRAs are among the safest central nervous system drugs prescribed by doctors, and that they are effective in short-term treatment of insomnia. The FDA has approved all of these drugs for short-term use (about four weeks or less). Several are also FDA-approved for long-term use because studies have shown them to be safe and effective when used for six months or more.

While many people worry that prescription sleep aids are habit-forming, researchers offer a reassuring picture. Studies show that people with insomnia do not tend to abuse sleep aids. People who stop taking BzRA hypnotics rarely experience physical withdrawal symptoms other than rebound insomnia, which can occur if you abruptly stop taking one of the shorter-acting hypnotics. Generally, rebound insomnia only lasts one or two nights and can be avoided by gradually tapering the dose over a few nights. Of course, it is also possible that you will continue to sleep poorly once you stop taking hypnotics if the original underlying cause of your sleep problem has not been treated.

→ **Around 1300 B.C. in ancient Egyptian times, opium was widely offered as a treatment to relieve insomnia.**

SLEEPWALKING, SLEEP EATING, AND OTHER STRANGE SIDE EFFECTS OF HYPNOTICS

Almost all medications have some risk of side effects and hypnotics are no different. Among people who report side effects, the most common ones are next-day grogginess (hangover), dizziness, headaches, and forgetfulness. These side effects tend to occur more often in people who use higher doses and longer-acting hypnotics, and in people who are taking medications for other health conditions. Older adults in particular may be at risk because they may be more sensitive to the effects of medications and may be taking other medications. Older adults waking up at night after taking a sleeping pill may be at risk of falling. Lowering the dose or switching to a different hypnotic can relieve side effects in many cases, so it is important to talk with your healthcare provider to help you get the best results.

While most patients tolerate the FDA-approved sleeping pills well, there have been a few cases of sleepwalking, sleep eating, and sleep driving in people taking them. This is an uncommon reaction to the drug, but since these are potentially dangerous behaviors, it is important to know some of the risk factors and talk about them with your doctor before starting treatment. Risk factors include taking medium to high doses, being female, having multiple medical or psychiatric disorders, taking multiple medications, and having untreated restless legs syndrome. However, only a small number of people treated with sleeping pills will develop these weird sleep behaviors.

TIPS ON TAKING PRESCRIPTION SLEEP MEDICATIONS

→ **Taking a prescribed sleep aid requires knowledge about how to use it safely.**

- Ask your doctor what medication is being prescribed and whether it is an FDA-approved hypnotic, what side effects might occur, when to take the medication, and how long it will be used.

- Use the medication according to the dose and length of time your doctor recommends.

- Tell your doctor about any other medications you may be taking.

- Do not use alcohol while taking sleep aids.

- If you take a longer-acting sleep aid, make sure you allow enough time for a full night's sleep.

- When you first start taking a sleep aid, be careful doing activities that require next-day alertness (driving a car, operating machinery, etc.) until you know how you are affected the morning after taking a sleep aid.

- NEVER use someone else's prescribed medication!

WHO MAY BE AT RISK TAKING SLEEP AIDS?

+ People who snore or who have sleep apnea: breathing may be further impaired. Ramelteon is an exception—it does not affect breathing in people with obstructive sleep apnea.
+ Individuals who drink alcohol: taking pills with alcohol increases the effects of both.
+ The elderly, and anyone who needs to get up during the night: the sedating effects of hypnotics increase the risk of falling.
+ Those who have to drive or operate machinery soon after waking up: in longer-acting hypnotics, the risk of accidents may be increased.
+ Anyone who is "on call" during the night: it may be difficult to make important decisions, drive, care for children, or do other activities while hypnotics are still active in your body.
+ Pregnant women: most pregnant women should not use these drugs, so if you are pregnant, talk to your doctor about alternate options.

As with any medication, the particular drug prescribed for sleep problems will depend on the patient's diagnosis, age, health conditions, other medications being taken, and lifestyle. Work with your healthcare provider to find the treatment plan that works for you.

OTHER DRUGS: ANTIDEPRESSANTS, ANTIPSYCHOTICS, AND ANTIHISTAMINES

While a number of medications other than hypnotics are used by doctors to treat insomnia, approved hypnotics are usually preferred by sleep specialists because there is much more scientific evidence to support their use in treating sleep problems. Antidepressants, antipsychotics, antihistamines, and other drugs are sometimes considered as alternatives, but their effectiveness for treating sleep problems has not been extensively studied. These drugs can also have significant side effects, so it is important to talk with your doctor before taking a medication.

ANTIDEPRESSANTS AND OTHER DRUGS USED TO TREAT MENTAL DISORDERS

The FDA has not approved the use of these drugs for the treatment of insomnia and thus they are used "off-label." Some studies have shown that antidepressants, such as trazodone and doxepin, can improve sleep when prescribed for short-term use. It is less clear how effective antidepressants are for long-term treatment of insomnia, and there is little data showing how well they work in non-depressed individuals. Antidepressants act through different parts of the brain than hypnotics do, and there is wide variation in their sleep effects. For insomnia, some doctors prescribe the "off-label" use of drugs normally used to treat serious psychiatric conditions such as schizophrenia because a side effect of these products is sleepiness. Since drugs used for psychiatric problems can have significant side effects there may be safety concerns, so it is important to discuss these concerns with your doctor.

ANTIHISTAMINES

The main ingredient in over-the-counter (OTC) sleeping aids such as Tylenol PM®, Advil PM®, Unisom®, and Sominex® is an antihistamine, which acts on a different part of the brain than prescription hypnotics do. There is not much published research on the use of these medications as a treatment for insomnia and they should not be taken for longer than the directions indicate (usually a few days to two weeks). If your sleep problems persist, it is important to talk with your doctor to identify the underlying cause and determine the best treatment plan.

It is also important to pay attention to your body's physical response to OTC sleep aids. For example, antihistamines may help you sleep at night, but you may also have a "sleep hangover" the following morning. Other side effects can include dizziness, lack of coordination, forgetfulness, blurred vision, and trouble with mental alertness the following day. Even though these drugs are generally safe and not habit-forming, you should consult your doctor before taking them if you have other health conditions (such as breathing problems or glaucoma) or are taking other medications. As with hypnotics, OTC sleep aids should not be used if you are also taking alcohol or other drugs with sedating effects. Older people should be especially cautious because their slower metabolisms can mean that these drugs stay in the body longer and can then cause daytime sleepiness. Women who are pregnant or nursing should also talk with a doctor before starting any type of OTC sleep treatment.

MELATONIN AND HERBAL REMEDIES

There is a myth that the "natural" dietary supplements and herbal remedies that are sold to promote sleep are somehow safer and more effective than prescription medications. There is no strong scientific evidence at this time to support their safety and effectiveness in treating sleep problems.

Herbal products and nutritional supplements (such as melatonin) are not required to undergo the same rigorous testing that drugs must go through in order to be legally sold. Therefore, their side effects and long-term impact are often not known. In addition, since the manufacturing of these products is not regulated by the FDA, they can vary in their concentrations and may contain other ingredients that can cause health problems.

MELATONIN

Melatonin is a naturally occurring hormone secreted by the pineal gland, a small gland in the center of the brain. Melatonin's secretion is controlled by the light-dark cycle, which is a key part of the system regulating sleep and your body clock. Bright light prevents the release of melatonin, so levels of melatonin are much higher at night. This has earned melatonin the nickname "Dracula of hormones," since it only comes out in the dark. Because melatonin is a natural part of the human sleep-wake cycle, many people think that by taking it as a pill, it will help them fall asleep faster or stay asleep longer.

This may be true, but more research is needed to determine whether melatonin is an effective treatment for insomnia. In some studies, people taking melatonin reported that they fell asleep faster and had better sleep quality, although melatonin's effects on the ability to stay asleep throughout the night are less consistent. There is stronger evidence that melatonin is useful for treating circadian rhythm disorders, such as jet lag, that cause our internal body clock to be out of sync with daily activities and schedules. Several studies suggest that taking melatonin close to the target bedtime at your destination, starting on the day of travel and continuing for several days, reduces the length of time it takes to get on a normal sleep pattern at your destination. More studies, however, are needed to confirm these findings and to determine the best doses of melatonin to use. In addition to alleviating jet lag, melatonin may also help people who work irregular shifts and need to adjust their schedules. When taken in low doses at the appropriate time, some studies show that melatonin can help advance or delay the sleep-wake cycle.

> In addition to alleviating jet lag, melatonin may also help people who work irregular shifts and need to adjust their schedules.

Melatonin is thought to be safe for short-term use—it is not addictive and has few known side effects—but there is not yet evidence on whether long-term use is safe and effective. The most commonly reported side effects are fatigue, dizziness, irritability, headaches, and confusion. Since there are risks of daytime sleepiness, it is important to be careful driving or operating machinery after taking melatonin. There have not been any reported cases of proven toxicity or overdose from melatonin use. However, certain individuals should take extra caution when using melatonin. People with blood clotting disorders or who are taking blood-thinning medications should talk with a doctor before using melatonin. Patients with type 1 diabetes should also be careful, since low doses of melatonin can cause reduced glucose tolerance and insulin sensitivity. In some cases, melatonin has also been shown to cause a drop in blood pressure so individuals already taking medications to lower blood pressure should be especially careful. Since melatonin is a hormone, women who are pregnant or attempting to become pregnant should also avoid taking it. These are important concerns that highlight the need for more research on long-term safety in humans.

Why is melatonin available without a prescription?

You've probably seen melatonin in stores or in advertisements. No other hormone is available in the United States without a prescription. Because melatonin is contained naturally in some foods, it can be sold as a dietary supplement, just like vitamins and minerals, without being approved by the FDA or controlled in the same way as drugs. Because it is not categorized as a drug, synthetic melatonin can be made in factories that are not regulated by the FDA. Side effects do not have to be listed on the product's packaging. The listed doses may not be controlled or accurate, so the amount of melatonin in a pill you take may not be the same as the amount listed on the package. If you are thinking about taking melatonin, these are some of the risks you should consider.

For melatonin to be helpful, the dosage and time of day it is taken must be appropriate for the sleep problem. Taking it at the wrong time of day can reset your biological clock in the wrong direction. So, even though melatonin is available without a prescription, it helps to talk with your healthcare provider before taking it to figure out if it is really the best way to resolve your sleep problems.

L-TRYPTOPHAN

L-tryptophan is an amino acid that has been studied as a hypnotic. The evidence for its effectiveness in treating insomnia is limited, and is based on studies with small numbers of people. In studies, some people have reported reduced time to fall asleep and improved sleep quality, but the evidence is inconclusive. Better research is needed to determine whether L-tryptophan is an effective sleep aid.

Concerns have also been raised about its possible toxic effects, especially when used in combination with certain psychiatric medications.

> → **Many people know that turkey contains L-tryptophan, but so do these other foods: chocolate, oats, bananas, mangoes, dried dates, milk, yogurt, cottage cheese, red meat, eggs, fish, other poultry, sesame, chickpeas, sunflower seeds, pumpkin seeds, spirulina, and peanuts.**

HERBAL REMEDIES

Right now, there is not sufficient scientific knowledge on the effectiveness and safety of herbal treatments for insomnia. Like melatonin, herbal remedies do not have to go through the rigorous research studies and FDA regulations that prescription drugs do, so there is less data available on their effects on sleep and their interactions with other drugs and medical conditions.

Be smart about what you put into your body. The fact that herbal products come from plants and are advertised as "natural" does not mean they are "natural" for the human body. The main issue is that herbal products and supplements don't have to be tested to prove they work well and are safe before they're sold. The herbal products you buy also may not be pure—they are not required to be tested for manufacturing consistency, so they may contain other ingredients, such as plant pollen, that could make you sick if you have certain health problems or allergies. Many herbal products can cause side effects and can change the way prescription or OTC drugs work in your body. For example, some herbal supplements can change the way your body absorbs certain drugs, so that even if you take the right amount of your medication, it won't be absorbed at high enough levels to help the condition it is prescribed to treat. This can cause serious problems. Talk to your doctor before taking herbal products, particularly if you have existing health conditions or are taking medications.

> The main issue is that herbal products and supplements don't have to be tested to prove they work well and are safe before they're sold.

Let's take a look at some of the herbal supplements that are most widely claimed to promote sleep.

Valerian

Of all the herbal supplements listed here, valerian is the most extensively studied for its effectiveness in promoting sleep. Valerian is a root that can be steeped in boiling water for tea, and it is also sold in capsules, tablets, and liquid extracts. In some studies, it has been shown to reduce the time it takes to fall asleep and improve sleep quality. Other studies have shown that it has little or no effect on sleep, so the evidence remains inconclusive and it cannot be recommended widely as a sleep aid yet. Side effects of valerian are reported to be few and mild, and include headaches, weakness, dizziness, and morning sleepiness. Some studies indicate that ongoing nightly use may be more effective than a single dose, with increasing effects over four weeks. Research suggests that valerian is generally safe to use for short periods of time (four to six weeks), but no information is available on the long-term safety of valerian.

Kava

Kava is a root that is used in beverages, extracts, capsules, tablets, and topical solutions. While scientific studies provide some evidence that kava is beneficial for treating anxiety, with improvements over one to four weeks, it is not a proven therapy for sleep problems. Side effects of short-term, light use may include an upset stomach, rash, mild headaches, and drowsiness. Chronic or heavy use has been associated with skin disorders, abnormal muscle movements, kidney damage, seizures, and blood abnormalities. The FDA has issued a warning that kava has been linked to a risk of liver damage, but it is not clear what dose or duration is associated with a risk of liver damage. It is also not clear what other factors may have contributed to the reported liver damage in people who experienced problems, so in general, caution is warranted. Because this product has uncertain effectiveness and may have lethal side effects, it has been removed from the market in some countries.

St. John's Wort

St. John's Wort is an herb used to make teas and tablets with concentrated extracts. Research shows it can be effective in treating mild to moderate depression, but there is not yet enough evidence to recommend it for sleep disorders. Side effects are not common, but the ones most often observed are an upset stomach, skin reactions, fatigue, anxiety, sexual dysfunction, dizziness, headaches, and dry mouth. In studies, St. John's Wort has been well-tolerated at its recommended doses for one to three months.

Lavender

Lavender is a plant that is often taken for anxiety, restlessness, and insomnia, and is most commonly used in aromatherapy. Dried lavender flowers can also be used to make teas or liquid extracts to be taken by mouth. There is currently little scientific evidence of lavender's effectiveness in treating sleep problems, and studies so far suggest a small overall effect on anxiety. In some cases, drowsiness has been reported after lavender aromatherapy or consuming lavender teas or extracts. Side effects, while not common, can include headaches, changes in appetite, nausea, and confusion. However, because lavender is often used in conjunction with behaviors that may lead to relaxation (for example, a warm bath), it may be helpful in initiating sleep in some patients. Try using the lavender bath salts in this kit to relax before bedtime.

Drowsiness has been reported after lavender aromatherapy or consuming lavender teas or extracts.

Chamomile

Chamomile is a plant whose leaves can be consumed as a tea, liquid extract, capsule, or tablet, and can be used in aromatherapy or applied to the skin as a lotion or ointment. It is often used to promote sleep and relieve anxiety. Since chamomile has not been widely studied, there is little evidence to support its effectiveness for treating sleep problems. Side effects include reports of rare allergic reactions, such as skin rashes, throat swelling, and shortness of breath. A person is more likely to experience an allergic reaction to chamomile if he or she is also allergic to related plants in the daisy family, including ragweed, chrysanthemums, marigolds, and daisies. Chamomile can cause drowsiness, so caution should be used when driving or operating machinery. Overall, though, better research is needed before a conclusive recommendation can be made on chamomile.

Passion flower

Passion flower, which can be taken as a dried herb in tea, is traditionally used as a sedative and hypnotic for insomnia. Some studies suggest it causes drowsiness, but there is not sufficient research evidence to support its therapeutic value in people with insomnia. Some allergies have been reported, such as hypersensitivity reactions in skin, but passion flower is generally considered to be safe, with few side effects. Some side effects, such as rapid heart rate, nausea, and vomiting have been reported, but this may have been due to contaminants.

IS MEDICATION RIGHT FOR ME?

It is important to talk with your doctor before taking any of these herbal supplements, especially if you have an existing medical condition or are taking other drugs. Women who are pregnant or nursing should not take any of these supplements without medical advice, because risks to the fetus or infant have not been evaluated, and some of these products, such as chamomile, may act as a uterine stimulant or lead to miscarriage.

To sum up, there are many options for treating sleep problems—prescription sleep aids, over-the-counter drugs, and dietary and herbal supplements. It's always best to talk with your doctor before embarking on a new treatment, so that you can make sure he or she has diagnosed the root cause of your sleep problems and find a treatment plan tailored to your individual needs. Often behavioral treatments may be what you need and not any medication or supplement. If you have persistent sleep problems, a combination of prescription medications and behavioral treatments may provide the best results for managing your sleep. You can find more information on this in the following chapter and by visiting the National Sleep Foundation's Web site at www.sleepfoundation.org.

+ Chapter 8 +

Tips for
Better Sleep

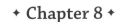

THE KEY TO SLEEPING WELL for life is developing and practicing good sleep habits. Unfortunately, many people learn poor sleep habits early in life that make it difficult to prevent and overcome sleep difficulties as they occur. Some people turn to medications to treat sleep troubles, but behavioral remedies are often more effective, especially for treating sleep problems for the long-term. There are a number of behavioral approaches to sleep challenges and this chapter covers some of the most popular, including good sleep habits, nutritional concerns, and cognitive behavioral therapy. The following are methods of developing good sleep habits that everyone should practice, whether they currently have sleep problems or not. But first...

THE MATTRESS MATTERS

And so does the pillow. It is difficult to fall asleep and stay asleep if your bed and pillow are uncomfortable or cause pain. While exhausted people can sleep almost anywhere, including park benches and airport floors, for regular nightly use a quality mattress and pillow are crucial.

There are a variety of mattress types for sale and it is important for you to find the best one for your needs. Mattresses can be filled with air, foam, cotton, synthetic materials, springs, and even horsehair, and they come in varying degrees of hardness. Although it seems obvious that the surface you sleep on is critical to your quality of sleep, there is still very little research on the topic. Old research indicated that a firm mattress was best, but new studies suggest that for people with lower back pain a medium-firm mattress results in less pain at night and in the daytime. One recent trend has been for people to purchase softer mattresses, often with "pillow tops."

The bottom line is that each person has to detect their own comfort level. If you wake up with pain in your shoulders, hips, or back that you didn't have when you went to sleep, it might be time to think about getting a new mattress. A two-minute test in a store may not be enough to determine what type of mattress is best for you, so be sure the store has a return policy if it turns out to be uncomfortable.

> → **In the sixteenth and seventeenth centuries, mattresses were generally stuffed with straw or down and placed atop a lattice-work of rope. The expression "sleep tight" comes from this time period, when the ropes needed regular tightening to be firm.**

USE THE BEDROOM ONLY FOR SLEEP AND SEX

This commandment can be challenging in communities where housing is expensive and people have all their belongings in one or two rooms. But, the point is that the bedroom should not contain a blaring television, a computer continuously on, or a fax machine spewing out paper at random times. There are two reasons for this. The first is that the various gadgets may actually wake you up. The second and possibly more important reason is that you may begin to associate your bedroom with everything but sleep. Your bedroom should be calm, quiet, and dark, and you should be able to control the temperature. In other words, it should be a shrine for sleep.

Your bedroom should be calm, quiet, and dark, and you should be able to control the temperature.

DEVELOP A RITUAL AT BEDTIME

Whether we know it or not, most people and many animals have a ritual that paves the way into sleep. A lion may circle its den several times before entering; a young child may have a bath and then have a bedtime story read to them before being tucked in; adults often have routines such as washing up, reading, fluffing their pillow just so, and getting comfortable in bed. They may read the same article in the same issue of *The New Yorker* for the thirtieth night in a row, falling asleep after the first paragraph. Establish your ritual. You may already have one. Just do it every night…

…AT THE SAME TIME

Your body, brain, and biological clock thrive on regularity. Try to go to bed at the same time every night and wake up the same time every morning, even during weekends and holidays. Changing these times results in some biological systems going haywire. Keeping a regular schedule synchronizes all these body functions and makes falling asleep easier.

DE-STRESS YOUR BRAIN

It is very important to avoid anything that will arouse your brain in the hour or two before going to sleep. Some examples of arousing activities that you should not do before bed are:

- ✦ Balancing your checkbook.
- ✦ Checking your investment portfolio.
- ✦ Watching exciting or upsetting television programs or news.
- ✦ Playing video games.
- ✦ Text messaging a friend or colleague.
- ✦ Having an argument.

It takes only seconds to have your brain aroused, but it may take hours to calm the brain down. The reason is that your body releases chemicals when your brain is aroused and it takes some time for the levels of these chemicals to drop. That is why it is essential to relax and wind down before going to bed.

GET OUT OF BED

This may seem odd coming from a sleep clinician, but many people with sleep problems spend way too much time in bed. If you do not fall asleep within twenty minutes, get up and do something else. Do not just lie there with your mind racing, playing back the day's events and trying to fall asleep. Most often, the harder you try to sleep, the more difficult and frustrating sleep becomes. That is because stress, frustration, and anger all result in the release of chemicals that arouse your brain.

If you have trouble sleeping due to worry, preoccupation, or stress, the best thing to do is get out of bed and do something boring until you feel sleepy enough to go back to bed. Do not read an exciting book or article. Do not check to see whether there's a good movie on television. Another reason not to lie in bed awake is that you will create a negative sleep association. That is, your brain will begin to associate your bed with not sleeping. Then, you will climb into bed every night expecting not to sleep and, sure enough, you won't.

MAKE A LIST

Some people can't fall asleep because they are planning what they will be doing the next day and fretting that they will forget something. If you are one of these people, before you even get to bed, make a list of such things, and then put the list down. Keep the list in another part of the house—not next to your bed.

DON'T EXERCISE CLOSE TO BEDTIME

Physical activity and sleep are closely linked. For the most part, being active and getting regular exercise facilitates sleep and helps prevent sleep problems. However, don't expect to fall asleep right away after vigorous exercise (with one exception, see below). It is better to exercise earlier in the day than in the one to two hours before bed. Again, your body releases chemicals when you exercise and these natural "performance enhancing" chemicals degrade your ability to fall asleep and stay asleep. Except…

SEX IS OKAY

For reasons that are not well understood, sexual activity, even when vigorous, does not seem to interfere with the ability to fall asleep. It is very likely that the chemicals released during sexual activity are distinct from those released during other types of exercise.

WATCH WHAT YOU EAT

It is best not to eat anything immediately before going to bed because certain foods may cause heartburn, which can make it difficult to fall sleep. Heartburn symptoms may also occur several hours after eating, disrupting sleep later in the night, or symptoms may be "silent." That is, you may not be aware of them, but even silent heartburn can keep you awake. If heartburn is interfering with your sleep despite avoiding heartburn-causing foods, you may need a prescription medication that reduces the production of acid by your stomach. Taking antacids or milk at bedtime may only be a very temporary fix.

PUT AWAY THE CAFFEINE...

Caffeine, the most widely used stimulant, is a common sleep stealer. Consuming moderate amounts of caffeine (one to two servings per day) is usually not enough to keep most people from sleeping. However, excessive caffeine consumption or consuming caffeine late in the day can cause insomnia. If you are having trouble sleeping at night, avoid caffeine after lunchtime. Remember that it's not just coffee and tea that contain caffeine. Many other products, including the five hundred or so caffeine-infused drinks sold worldwide, may contain as much or more caffeine as a cup of coffee. In particular, energy drinks may contain more caffeine than even a cup of coffee. Such products comprise a $3.5 billion market, much of which is directed at children and young adults. Read the labels of these beverages. Compare their caffeine content to that of coffee, which usually contains 80 to 150 mg of caffeine. However, some coffee vendors sell very large cups that may contain double that amount of caffeine.

> Excessive caffeine consumption or consuming caffeine late in the day can cause insomnia.

...AND THE ALCOHOL

Alcohol is another commonly used sleep stealer. According to the National Sleep Foundation's 2005 Sleep in America Poll, 11 percent of Americans use alcohol to help them sleep at least a few nights a week. Alcohol is a sedative and may help you fall asleep initially. However, alcohol may cause sleep disruption later in the night. The drop in blood alcohol level that occurs after several hours has an arousing effect on the brain, which can disrupt sleep and make returning to sleep quite difficult. Another big downside of alcohol is that it makes snoring much worse. And because alcohol relaxes muscles, including those of the upper breathing passage, it may also cause people who snore to develop sleep apnea or worsen the condition in those who already have it.

CHECK THE MEDICATIONS YOU ARE TAKING

Many prescription and over-the-counter drugs can cause nighttime insomnia and/or daytime sleepiness. Read product labels to see if your medications, food, or herbal supplements have an effect on sleep. If a medication label says "non-drowsy," it may mean that it can keep you awake. Some non-drowsy medications may not affect your sleep (e.g., certain antihistamines), while others may contain ingredients that will keep you awake (e.g., certain cold medications). A caveat about health food products: in some countries there has been a recall of herbal supplements that helped people to fall asleep. They worked well. They worked too well. It turned out they contained chemicals found in sleeping pills!

IS YOUR DIET CAUSING SLEEP PROBLEMS?

Being mindful of nutrition is also a key to sleeping well. Certain diets, lifestyle choices, or medical conditions may result in nutritional deficiencies that cause sleep problems. For example, strict vegetarians can become deficient in iron and other nutrients such as vitamin B12 or folic acid. Low levels of these three nutrients can lead to restless legs syndrome and/or excessive movements in sleep, which can lead to insomnia.

> → **Some of history's most notable figures have been consummate nap-takers, including Leonardo da Vinci, Winston Churchill, and John F. Kennedy.**

Heavy menstrual cycles can also lead to iron deficiency, especially when the diet is poor or another cause of blood loss is present. Donating large amounts of blood may lead to iron deficiency, which may not be picked up by the finger prick test at the blood bank. Certain diseases may cause reduced iron or B12 stores. Some examples are conditions associated with decreased absorption from the intestinal tract and diseases that cause loss of iron. Also, people who have had bariatric surgery for obesity may not absorb some important nutrients. If you feel your sleep difficulty may be caused by nutritional deficiency, talk to your doctor about the problem.

NAPPING

Napping in adults is an indication of sleep deprivation, either due to not enough sleep or poor quality sleep. The one cure for sleep deprivation is sleep. Not caffeine. Not splashing water on your face. Not biting your lip. Not having cold air blow in your face while you drive to try to maintain alertness. Only sleep replaces sleep. If you are sleep deprived, a nap can be a wonderful lifesaver.

Here are some tips about naps that apply to most people: a nap that is one to three hours is too long. A nap should be short, usually anywhere between ten and forty-five minutes. A longer nap may leave you feeling groggy. A longer nap may also make it difficult for you to fall asleep at your normal bedtime.

MAKE SLEEP A PRIORITY

Many people believe that sleep is a waste of time and try to get along with the least amount of sleep possible. They drink copious amounts of coffee to try to maintain alertness during the day and use alarm clocks to wake up very early in the morning. Then, they complain about how rotten they feel all day and how much trouble they have falling asleep at night. These people tend to be very irritable and moody. They have not yet made the connection between how they feel and their sleep habits.

Sleep should be a priority for everyone. It is critical to your health. Once you are aware of your sleep-habits you can begin to change them if they are detrimental to your well-being.

TAKE A BEHAVIORAL APPROACH
TO SLEEP PROBLEMS

People with sleep problems are increasingly turning to cognitive behavioral therapy (CBT), a form of treatment that actively engages the individual in his or her own treatment. CBT works by changing the attitudes, beliefs, and behaviors that perpetuate illness. The underlying assumption of CBT is that individuals can learn how to resolve a problem themselves with the help of a therapist.

CBT is used to treat a range of issues and conditions, including:

✦ Anxiety

✦ Phobias

✦ Depression

✦ Substance abuse

✦ Weight management

COGNITIVE BEHAVIORAL THERAPY FOR SLEEP PROBLEMS

Though the basic principles of CBT are similar no matter which condition is being addressed, CBT has different components for different difficulties. For sleep problems, the goals of CBT are to:

+ Undo misconceptions about sleep.
+ Alleviate sleep-related anxiety.
+ Teach individuals how behavior affects sleep.
+ Establish healthy sleep habits for life.

HOW COGNITIVE BEHAVIORAL THERAPY FOR SLEEP PROBLEMS WORKS

With CBT for sleep problems, patients work with a therapist to create positive and lasting sleep associations. Some of the most common components of CBT for sleep problems include:

+ Cognitive restructuring
+ Sleep restriction
+ Stimulus control
+ Relaxation
+ Sleep habits

RELEARN HOW TO SLEEP

Cognitive restructuring targets the beliefs and attitudes that perpetuate sleep problems and teaches people how and why the sleep problems occur. For example, some people with sleep problems may worry excessively about how much sleep they are getting, which in turn makes it more difficult to sleep.

Through cognitive restructuring, patients learn to reduce or eliminate such worry to get the sleep they need.

SETTING LIMITS

For the sleep restriction component of CBT for sleep problems, a person's time in bed is limited to the amount of time he or she typically sleeps, and then gradually increased as sleep time increases. For example, if an individual normally spends ten hours in bed each night, but only sleeps for six of those hours, his or her time in bed would be limited to six hours. Using sleep restriction, the individual may initially sleep less than they did before beginning treatment. As sleep time begins to match time spent in bed, a strong association between the bed and sleep is formed.

TAKE SLEEP STEALERS OUT OF THE BEDROOM

Stimulus control is another very powerful component of CBT for sleep problems. It involves identifying and eliminating all potential "sleep stealers" in and around one's bed and bedroom. For example, many people with sleep problems are clock watchers, agonizing over every minute they are awake and dreading the coming day for the sleepiness it will bring. For these people, the only way to end the nightly clock obsession is to take it out of the bedroom or at least turn the clock so it can't be seen during the night.

Other sleep stealers include:
+ Televisions
+ Electronic games
+ Fax machines
+ Computers

In some cases, stimulus control requires sleeping apart from a spouse or other bed partner if he or she snores, has another sleep problem, or gets up during the night. This can be very difficult, but it doesn't have to be permanent. Sleep problems can be treated and nighttime disruptions can be reduced or eliminated. For example, if one member of a couple gets up earlier than the other, he or she can take steps to avoid waking his or her bed partner.

Stimulus control may also target pets. It is amazing that people allow their pets to come between them and their sleep, but it happens often. Over the years many sleep professionals have seen and heard it all:

+ Cats that sleep in the bed and wrestle with their owner's feet all night long.
+ Dogs that wander in and out of the bedroom.
+ Snoring bulldogs.
+ Caged birds that never quiet down.

It is essential to develop a strategy that keeps your pet from interfering with your sleep, and that may mean banishing it from the bedroom entirely. Do not go to your healthcare provider with complaints of trouble sleeping when the problem is your pet, especially if you've decided in advance never to change your rules about where the pet is allowed.

Stimulus control also includes getting out of bed if sleep does not come easily (e.g., within twenty minutes). As discussed earlier in this chapter, it is better to get up and engage in a relaxing (and preferably boring) activity and then return to bed only when sleepy. Ultimately, stimulus control allows the person to re-associate the bed and bedroom with sleep.

RELAX THE MIND AND BODY

Relaxation therapy may also be prescribed by a CBT therapist for sleep problems. There are many different relaxation techniques that can be employed, and the choice of which to try may depend on patient preference. Some examples of relaxation strategies are:

+ Yoga
+ Pilates
+ Meditation
+ Massage
+ Progressive muscle relaxation
+ Breathing exercises

LEARN THE FUNDAMENTALS OF SLEEP HABITS

Sleep habits are a critical component of CBT for sleep problems and for long-term sleep health. It refers to habits and lifestyle factors that may affect sleep and alertness. A CBT therapist may create a list of "dos" and "don'ts" that are particular to each patient, but the fundamentals of sleep habits are the same for everyone. They include the tips and strategies covered in this chapter, including:

+ Maintain a regular sleep-wake cycle.
+ Establish a relaxing bedtime routine.
+ Create an ideal sleep environment.
+ Don't eat a heavy meal or exercise immediately before going to bed.
+ Limit caffeine.
+ Avoid alcohol.

THE BENEFITS OF COGNITIVE BEHAVIORAL THERAPY FOR SLEEP PROBLEMS

CBT for sleep problems may be conducted in a variety of settings, including one-on-one and group therapy. No matter how it is practiced, research suggests that even a few CBT sessions can significantly improve symptoms of insomnia, daytime sleepiness, and sleep anxiety. More importantly, these effects are generally long-lasting.

Some of the benefits of cognitive behavioral therapy for sleep problems include:

+ Patient involvement: patients and therapists work together to set goals and determine the duration of therapy.
+ Flexibility: CBT allows therapists the freedom to tailor treatment to each patient in a variety of settings.
+ Compatibility: CBT can be used in concert with medications and/or other forms of psychological and behavioral therapies.
+ Safety: CBT for insomnia carries no side effects or risk of dependency.

Evidence suggests that CBT is very effective at treating sleep problems and for preventing future insomnia. CBT may not be enough, however, to resolve sleep problems for everyone. In these cases, CBT may be used in combination with sleep medications and other strategies. Research suggests that using CBT in combination with medications and sleep habits is far more effective at treating insomnia in the long-term than medications alone.

GETTING STARTED WITH COGNITIVE BEHAVIORAL THERAPY FOR SLEEP PROBLEMS

You may consider CBT if you have sleep problems that persist for weeks or months despite careful attention to sleep habits. For many individuals, the main obstacle to CBT for sleep problems is locating a therapist who has experience in dealing with sleep problems. CBT is a relatively new treatment and practitioners may be difficult to find in some parts of the country. For more information on CBT for sleep problems, visit the National Sleep Foundation online at www.sleepfoundation.org.

In this chapter you learned that there are many things that you can do to improve your own sleep and the sleep of others without the use of any medications. You learned about the principles of sleep habits and how to apply them. In addition, there are excellent treatments available that do not require the use of any drugs, but do require the help of a healthcare professional.

IN CONCLUSION

We hope that now that you've come to the end of this book you have learned a great deal about the importance of sleep and about the many conditions that can impact your sleep. We hope that you have learned that although there are many problems someone might have with sleep, there are also many solutions that you and your doctor can use to improve your sleep. As your sleep improves, so will your health and well-being.

We wish you restful nights and days filled with energy. We hope that we have achieved our goal that you go to bed, shut your eyes, and drift off peacefully, waking up alert and in a great mood, ready to conquer your day. Sweet dreams!

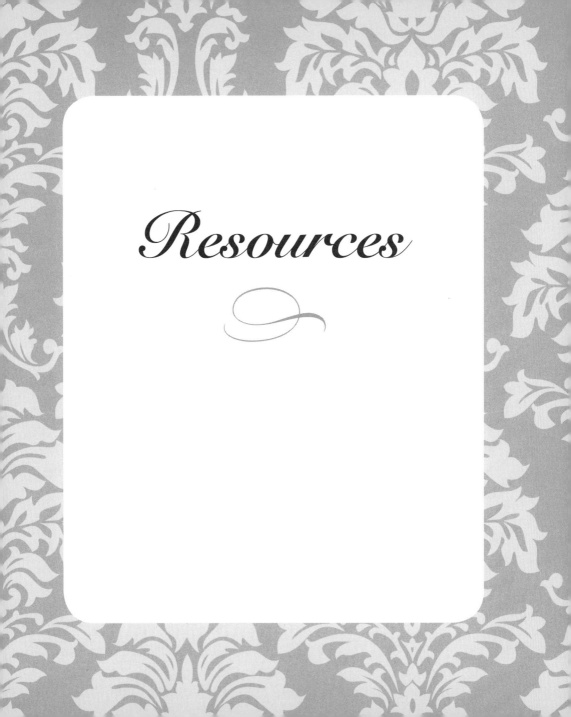

Resources

National Sleep Foundation
(for sleep information and a listing of sleep centers)
www.sleepfoundation.org
www.drowsydriving.org
www.sleepforkids.org

American Academy of Pediatrics
www.aap.org

American Academy of Dental Sleep Medicine
www.aadsm.org

American Academy of Sleep Medicine
www.aasmnet.org

American Lung Association
www.lungusa.org

American Sleep Apnea Association
www.sleepapnea.org

Centers for Disease Control and Prevention
www.cdc.gov/sleep

Mayo Clinic
www.mayoclinic.org

Narcolepsy Network
www.narcolepsynetwork.org

National Fibromyalgia Association
www.fmaware.org

National Institutes of Health

www.nih.gov

National Center for Alternative and Complementary Medicine
www.nccam.nih.gov

National Center on Sleep Disorders Research
www.nhlbi.nih.gov/about/ncsdr

National Heart, Lung, and Blood Institute
www.nhlbi.nih.gov

National Institute of Arthritis and Musculoskeletal Diseases
www.niams.nih.gov

National Institute of Child Health and Human Development
www.nichd.nih.gov

National Institute of Mental Health
www.nimh.nih.gov

National Institute of Neurological Disorders and Stroke
www.ninds.nih.gov

National Institute on Aging
www.nia.nih.gov

National Library of Medicine
www.nlm.nih.gov/medlineplus

National Organization for Rare Disorders

www.rarediseases.org

National Organizations for Youth Safety

www.noys.org

Restless Legs Syndrome Foundation

www.rls.org

Sleep Research Society

www.sleepresearchsociety.org

Index

INDEX

A

ADHD, 98–99

age and sleep, 22, 44–45, 61, 68, 72, 91–101, 104–13

alcohol, 50, 60, 69, 71, 82, 83, 88, 124, 125, 146

Alzheimer's disease, 110–111

antidepressants and antipsychotics, 125–126

antihistamines, 126–127

apnea. *See* sleep apnea

artificial light, 18

ASPS (advanced sleep phase syndrome), 71–73

awakeness, 18. *See also* sleepiness

B

babies and toddlers, 44, 94–96

bedwetting, 96, 97

behavioral remedies, 136, 149–155

Berlin Questionnaire (Modified), 55–57

body clock, 17, 18, 19, 24, 33, 72, 75–89, 106, 120, 128–129, 142

body functions during sleep, 16, 17–18, 19, 21, 58

brain and nervous system functions, 17–18, 52, 64, 68, 85

bruxism, 70–71

BzRAs (benzodiazepine receptor agonists), 119–123

C

caffeine, 84, 88, 145–146

cataplexy, 65, 66

central sleep apnea, 53

chamomile, 135

children and sleep, 91–101

chronotherapy, 72–73

circadian rhythms, 18, 33, 92, 106, 128

coffee, 76, 77, 148. *See also* caffeine

cognitive behavioral therapy (CBT). *See* behavioral remedies

co-morbid (secondary) insomnia, 36, 43

consequences
    of sleep deprivation, 12, 13, 16, 23, 25, 34, 85–86
    of sleep disorders, 42, 45, 49, 58

CPAP (continuous positive airway pressure), 59–60

D

Dement, Dr. William C., 13, 20

dreaming sleep. *See* REM sleep

drowsy driving, 34, 76–77

DSPS (delayed sleep phase syndrome), 71–72

E

Epworth Sleepiness Quiz, 30–32, 38

F

flying tips, 81–84

G

genetics, 54, 64–65

H

herbal remedies, 127–136

hyperarousal, 24, 44, 143

hypnotics, 72, 118–125

I

impact of medical conditions on sleep, 37–38, 42–43, 45

ineffective ways to stay awake, 88

insomnia, 24, 36–37, 42–48, 71, 72, 108–109, 147

internal clock. *See* body clock

J

jet lag, 77–84, 128

Johns, Dr. Murray, 30

K

kava, 133

Kleitman, Dr. Nathaniel, 20

L

lavender, 134

light, 18, 72–73, 81, 82

L–tryptophan, 130–131

M

mattress, 140–141

medical conditions and sleep, 37–38, 42–43, 45, 53, 61–62, 67, 105, 107–108

medications

    side effects of, 120, 122–24, 126–27, 129, 131–136

    and sleep, 43, 47, 63, 66, 68, 72, 107, 115–136, 147

melatonin, 17–18, 72, 81, 82, 107, 128–130

melatonin receptor agonists, 119–121

micro–sleep, 34

Mignot, Dr. Emmanuel, 65

multiple sleep latency test, 66

N

napping, 66, 67, 77, 88, 94–95, 105, 109, 147, 148

narcolepsy, 24, 64–67, 99, 109

nervous system functions, 17–18, 52, 64, 68, 85

nightmares, 67, 97

Non-REM sleep, 20

nutritional supplements.

    See herbal remedies

O

obesity, 49, 54, 59, 60, 99

obstructive sleep apnea. *See* sleep apnea

OTC (over the counter) sleep aids. *See* sleeping pills

P

paralysis during sleep, 19, 21, 65

partial arousal disorders. *See* sleepwalking

passion flower, 135

perpetuation, 37, 44

"Pickwickian syndrome," 52

polysomnography, 58

precipation, 37, 44

predisposition, 37, 44

prescription sleep aids. *See* sleeping pills

primary insomnia, 36

primary sleep disorders, 35–37

R

rebound insomnia, 120–21, 122–123

Rechtshaffen, Dr. Alan, 16

REM (rapid eye movement) sleep, 19–21, 64, 66

REM Sleep Behavior Disorder, 67–68

Restless Legs Syndrome, 36, 61–63, 99, 147

S

secondary (co–morbid) insomnia, 36, 43

shift work, 85–89, 128–129

side effects of medications, 120, 122–124, 126–127, 129, 131–136

SIDS (Sudden Infant Death Syndrome), 94

sleep and age, 22, 44–45, 91–101, 104–113

sleep

    amount needed, 21–23, 93

    apnea, 12, 23, 25, 48, 49, 51–61, 99, 108, 146

    architecture, 104–105, 106

    definition of, 16

deprivation, 12, 13, 16, 23, 25, 28, 32, 34
 consequences of, 12, 13, 16, 23, 25, 34, 69, 76–77
diary or log, 38
disorders, 12, 24, 28–73. *See also specific disorders*
 and age, 44–45, 53, 61, 68, 72, 107–109
 assessment of, 27–39
 frequency of, in population, 12, 28, 36, 42, 44–45, 53, 61, 64, 68, 72, 92, 105
 triggers of, 36–37
excessive, 22
habits, 35, 46, 47, 94, 140, 150, 153, 154
laboratory, 58–59
and medical conditions, 37–38, 42–43, 45, 53, 61–62, 67, 105, 107–108
and medications, 43, 47, 63, 66, 68, 72, 107, 115–136, 147
quality of, 22–23, 35–38
quantity of, 21–24, 32–33. *See also sleep deprivation*
reasons for, 16–17, 92
science of, 15–25
and shift work, 85–89, 128–129
slow wave, 20
stages of, 19–21, 104
timing of, 17–18
and travel, 76–84
Sleep Disorder Assessment Quiz, 39
sleep-promoting habits, 46, 86–88, 94, 96, 140–155
sleep stealers, 141, 151–152

sleep terror, 69, 98
sleep-wake cycle, 24, 84, 92
sleepiness, 18, 23, 28–32, 64, 66
sleeping pills, 47, 53, 60, 71, 81, 82, 108, 115–136
sleepwalking, 68–70, 98
snoring, 23, 35, 48–51, 146
Spielman, Dr. Art, 36
St. John's Wort, 134
stress, 70, 97, 101,143
suprachiasmatic nucleus, 17, 120
symptoms, 39, 96, 105. *See also specific disorders*

T
teenagers, 100–101
teeth-grinding, 70–71
"three P's," 36–37
tips for flying, 81–84
treatment
 of DSPS and ASPS, 72–73
 of insomnia, 46–48
 of REM Sleep Behavior Disorder, 67–68
 of Restless Legs Syndrome, 63
 of sleep apnea, 58–61
 of snoring, 50–51
 of teeth-grinding (bruxism), 71

V
valerian, 132–133

W
ways to stay awake, ineffective 88
women's issues, 36, 37–38, 45, 49, 108, 124, 125, 127, 136